TRUTH

The Ten Minute Life Plan

Ending Procrastination and Creating the Life You Want

From the TRUTH "How-To Series"

BILL CORTRIGHT

TRUTH: The Ten Minute Life Plan
Ending Procrastination and Creating the Life You Want
By Bill Cortright

Copyright © 2017 Bill Cortright

All rights reserved.

Transcendent Publishing
PO Box 66202
St. Pete Beach, FL 33736
www.transcendentpublishing.com

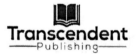

Second Edition April 2017 Transcendent Publishing

ISBN-10: 0-9987576-4-0
ISBN-13: 978-0-9987576-4-3

Library of Congress Control Number: 2017938477

Printed in the United States of America

To My Mom and Dad.

~Bill Cortright

TABLE OF CONTENTS

About the *TRUTH 'How-To'* Series

In 2009 I released the original book *The Stress-Response Diet* and I have lectured on its contents around the world. After selling over 150,000 copies, earlier this year I released *The NEW Stress-Response Diet and Lifestyle Program* which was the expanded and updated version. The sequel to my work with the Stress-Response Diet is *TRUTH: The Real Understanding to Health*. This book came out of the research I was doing to create a scientific based wellness program. The information that came out of those 5-years of trials was shocking as I will share, as the results were far more reaching than the wellness factors I was searching.

The *TRUTH 'How-To' Series* is a collection of short books that focus on particular areas that we need to develop in order to manage stress, create optimal health and create the life of our dreams. This book, *The Ten Minute Life Plan: Ending Procrastination and Creating the Life You Want*, is first in the *TRUTH* series.

Procrastination Tendencies

After three decades in the personal development field, if I have learned one thing it is that *tomorrow never comes*. When I was a young boy I was hurled into adulthood at a very early age. By the time I was twelve years old I had three paper routes and by the time I turned sixteen, I was living on my own, working and putting myself through high school. I was quite disciplined for my age as I had to handle many responsibilities. That did not mean I was organized or that I didn't procrastinate. In fact, I was the king of putting off today what could be done tomorrow, or even next week. If it wasn't for my best friend Mark bailing me out by doing ten art projects the day before they were due I would not have graduated high school. College wasn't any better as they actually didn't care if you went to class or not. That all changed once I joined the U.S. Navy because procrastination in the military is like a crime. What didn't change was my tendency to procrastinate. Over the years I developed systems that help people to take action toward their goals. I can now see why we put off the things we want the most in life. There are actual *scientific* reasons for why we procrastinate.

If you ask people why they procrastinate, you might possibly hear their real reasons. More than likely, though, you will hear their excuses. When an excuse sounds believable, it has a name—*rationalization*. It is its believability that makes rationalizing the original mind game. It's what you do in your thinking and feeling to explain away why your actions do not match up to your values and plans. It is the excuse you give yourself for your actions. It may seem reasonable but it *does not reflect the real reason*. In this **TRUTH How-To** book, **The Ten Minute Life Plan,** we will explore the real reasons we actually procrastinate. How diet, exercise, self-talk, childhood programs, and stress will cause us to procrastinate. More importantly I am going to give you easy-to-use tools that will help you break through and break out! Here is a list of a few procrastination tendencies.

If you have any of these then this simple book is about to change your life.

- Do you have a tendency to put things off to the point you must rush around in a panic mode to complete them?

- Do you have a tendency to daydream about what you are going to do one day, but never do it?

- Do you have a tendency to get lost with distractions such as computer games, social media, television, movies, etc.?

- Do you have a tendency to start a new diet every year? Do you fall off a diet the moment it does not meet your expectations?

- Do you lose weight and gain weight on a regular cycle? Are you overweight? Do you have a tendency to act impulsively without giving a second thought about the consequences of your actions? Do you choose immediate gratification and then feel guilty later?

- Do you have a tendency, during stressful events, to indulge in overeating especially sweets? Do you use any substances to deal with stress?

- Do you have a tendency to make to-do lists that never seems to get done? Do you feel overwhelmed with so much to do but get little accomplished?

- Do you have a tendency to overestimate your ability to get something done in a timely manner? Do you find yourself in the habit of extending deadlines?

- Do you have a tendency to set the same New Year's Resolutions year after year?

- Do you have a tendency to believe that there is a "magic time" that things will get done? Do you put off what you should do now with a set time in your head for when you will make up for the lost time?

If you answered yes to any of these questions, I have written this book specifically for *you.*

FREE BONUS!

As my gift to you, I've created a free course, *Living in the Green Zone,* consisting of five videos that take you through each of the **Five Life Categories: Career, Finance, Health, Relationships, Personal/Spiritual Development.** Each category has its own video packed with information and tips to live in the Green Zone.

This course is absolutely free to everyone who has purchased this book. Simply visit:

www.LivingRightWithBillCortright.com/10-minute-book

Introduction

You gotta make a change. It's time for us as a people to start making some changes; let's change the way we eat, let's change the way we live, and let's change the way we treat each other. You see, the old way wasn't working so it's on us, to do what we gotta do to survive.

—Tupac Shakur

I have developed my personal development programs and principles over the last thirty years while coaching clients on wellness and self-improvement from around the world, motivating people to live their best lives. I have found that there are ten principles that become the keys to personal development success. It doesn't matter what you want to change—from losing weight to making more money to building a strong relationship or creating a spiritual practice, it comes down to one key and that is the ability to take action and *do the work*. In my new book, *TRUTH*, I reveal the science of self-discipline and the success principles I have developed to create consistent action. To grow we must understand *procrastination* and why we put things off. We must understand why we sabotage ourselves, and we need tools that will keep us on track to do the work that is needed to create change.

There are three key elements that foster change.

- One, having a *strong purpose* to create the WHY factor
- Two, knowing exactly *what you want* with a clear vision
- Three, the management of the *stress response*

My focus has changed over the years of research and practical implications of my programs. In the beginning it was about creating a real weight loss program that would yield permanent results. Let's face

1

the facts. Every diet in the world will create weight loss. I rode that diet roller coaster many years before I created the *Five Links* back in 1985. I always tell people that my success isn't about me losing 100 pounds—it's about me maintaining that weight loss for 33 years. My body transformation from "fat kid" to bodybuilding champion was a great accomplishment but the greater accomplishment was the change within me that took me from a failure to a success. This is the change that propels me to fight all odds to create a life of purpose where I can live by my rules. It's this change that has allowed me to keep the 100 pounds off and to keep improving myself even though I am now in my fifties.

Every day I meet people that ask me the secret to discipline and creating change. They want to lose weight, increase their income, improve their relationships and find happiness. They all want to know the secret to living their life with a distinct purpose, with passion and energy that makes each day special. More important they want to know my secrets to being so disciplined. *My answer to this question is rather simple: Just Do It!* It seems Nike has had it right all these years. Change means you have to change your current habits and actions to get the results that you want. Sounds simple and it is, but that doesn't mean it's easy.

In *TRUTH*, I reveal a series of principles that I use to increase self-discipline, self-control and put an end to procrastination. The *Ten Minute Life Plan* is straight out of the tool chest of my Stress Mastery 'Shift Coaching' and the title of my book: The Seven Steps to Stress Mastery and the *TRUTH* book. This *TRUTH How-To* book will give you a dozen techniques to begin making the changes that you seek by conquering the tendency to procrastinate.

I am writing the *TRUTH* book out of my frustration of watching clients fail because they cannot get out of their own way. In other words, they sabotage themselves from attaining what they said they wanted. Over the last thirty years I have perfected the art of testing and resetting the individual metabolism. I have watched clients lose hundreds of pounds, get off medications and completely transform their body and lives, only to self-sabotage their efforts down the road and gain it all back. I have seen people who suffer day in and day out with health problems that we can reverse with simple lifestyle changes. Instead of taking action, they would rather wait to start a program that would change their life forever…but they *procrastinate*. I have also coached clients that will repeatedly sabotage their relationships, business ventures, basically anything that would make their life better. Why? Out of that simple question is why I wrote *TRUTH* and the *TRUTH How-To Series*.

So, how can I save money when everything I make goes straight to the bills? How can I lose weight when there is no time in my busy schedule to exercise or eat right? How can I live my dreams, write my book and climb Mt. Everest when I have to work? How can I invest in myself when I barely get by on the money I make? How can I start my own business without funding, experience or education? How can I find true love after age fifty? How can I be happy when the world is falling apart? *How can I change?* The answer is still the same. In order to change *you* have to change. If you keep doing the same things day after day, year after year, then you will live a life of regrets.

Change requires action and doing the work needed to create the result we want. We must beat procrastination.

In *The Ten Minute Life Plan* I will give you a dozen techniques that will turn on the self-discipline response and end procrastination in ten minutes or less. These are techniques I have used for the last thirty years and are now backed by the science of self-discipline. *The Ten Minute Life Plan* techniques will keep you moving forward toward whatever it is you desire. In other words, the techniques will help you to do the work.

It is very important that you understand why we self-sabotage. I will give you a quick overview of our survival DNA and how managing the survival responses will cause us to either move forward or run away from our goals. In my new book, *The Seven Steps to Stress Mastery*, I will take you on a journey through the science and spirituality of stress management. *The Ten Minute Life Plan* will give you that jump-start toward your new life with a dozen techniques that will turn on the *Action Response* in ten minutes or less. Action, action, action is the only secret to success.

My *Rocky* Story

It had long since come to my attention that people of accomplishment rarely sat back and let things happen to them. They went out and happened to things.   — Leonardo da Vinci

In my last book, *The NEW Stress-Response Diet*, I told of my story of climbing up and down on the weight scale and how I finally lost the weight and became a bodybuilding champion. There was a section in that story called "Finding the Power" about the moment the switch turned on and changed my life forever. I will relate the story here as told in that book.

Finding the Power

After spending more than a decade on the weight-loss roller coaster, my final ride would come as I entered my twenties. I was at the end of another diet cycle, which means I was in the process of gaining my weight back. I had gained back a hundred-plus pounds; I weighed over 270 pounds and was now wearing a tight size 48 pants (all at five feet six inches in height). I had been laid off my first real job as an adult. The stress of being unemployed and a life with zero direction was just too much. I began eating out of control and was drinking heavily on a daily basis. I then fell into a deep depression, and everything seemed hopeless.

My compulsive eating had completely deteriorated my life. I wouldn't leave my house for days while eating and drinking out of control. After several months of this behavior, I finally hit rock bottom. I was contemplating suicide when I received an absolute miracle that changed my life forever.

I stumbled upon a book that would set my life on a totally new course, a course I still follow today, twenty-five years later. The book was **The Power of Positive Thinking** *by Norman Vincent Peale. I had read all the diet and exercise books on the market, but I had never read*

anything like this. I can safely say this one book is the reason I'm here with you today. I can also say it's the reason I never gained that weight back and why I became successful in my field and my endeavors. It changed the most important element when it comes to weight loss and health; it changed my attitude and how I viewed the world. This is more powerful than any diet or type of exercise. For the first time in my life, I discovered the personal power of positive thinking. Years later, I would learn the power the mind actually had on the body's stress response.

I read the entire book in one day; I literally could not put it down. I felt a sense of empowerment and unbelievable hope, something I had never felt in the past. Then I simply took action. I started to move again; I would go out for leisurely walks. I started by going around the block. It didn't seem like much, but this was the first step of my new life and a lifestyle that I haven't stopped living for over twenty-five years now. I created a new state of mind; I believed I could do anything. I got rid of all the junk food I had been consuming and started eating sensibly. When it came to the exercise, that little walk around the block turned into two to three hours of walking daily! Over the next six months, I dropped over 125 pounds.

Along with the weight loss came a new attitude. In the past, I had lost weight, but never had changed my entire self-image. This time, I wasn't the fat person with the thin body; I was dynamic, outgoing, and extremely confident. Yes, I looked different, but the biggest difference was that I felt different. I have worked with thousands of people over the years, teaching them the truth about losing weight and getting healthy. I can tell you that when they get this feeling I'm describing— that extreme self-confidence, a sense of knowing they are changed from the inside—they will always get results. I will be giving you the tools to get this feeling; it's the key to any type of accomplishment, especially weight loss.

I wrote that more than five years ago and if you read it carefully the secret to all personal development is written in three words. ***"I took action…"*** Those three little words changed my life forever. Here is the part of the story that was not in the book. I always wanted two distinct things in life. One, I wanted to be in great shape and have the body of a god. Two, I wanted to be a super-hero.

In 1976 I sat in a movie theater and saw my inner hero on the screen, *Rocky*. Sylvester Stallone's movie made a huge impression on me. That movie made me believe that it didn't matter where I came from; that if I worked hard and was a good person I could be a champion.

The day after I saw Rocky I was up at 5a.m. ready to change my life. I gulped down three raw eggs, put on my sweat suit and started outside to go for a run. There was a hill in my neighborhood called Wilson's Hill and I was ready to attack it with everything I had. At that time, I was fifteen years old and probably 250 pounds of determination. The results weren't very Rocky-like as I only made it a third of the way up before getting violently sick and losing the eggs I had just chugged down.

I wish I could tell you that I sucked it up and attacked that damn Wilson's Hill again and again until I defeated it, but that would be a lie. I quit and it would be about twenty diets later and five more years before I lost weight and became that champion. *I became a master at self-sabotage and procrastination.* I did not attain success until I read the *Power of Positive Thinking* and only then was I able to change. I changed the way I talked, the way I walked, the way I thought, along with my entire attitude. After thirty years of coaching I know for a fact that change must come first in the mind before we see the effects in real life. Once we change our mind then we can—and will—change our actions.

The past few years I have been studying more about brain science and the science behind self-discipline. I have discovered that with precision we can create a life that will drive us toward what we really want. In my book *TRUTH* I offer a complete blueprint to creating a life of action while overcoming the resistance of procrastination. In my how-to book *The Ten Minute Life Plan* I will give you an overall explanation of why we do, or don't do, the things we need to do to change our life toward a life of prosperity and wellness. *The Ten Minute Life Plan* is an easy how-to guide to help you break through procrastination.

Chapter One: The Tale of Three Minds

Your subconscious never sleeps. It is always on the job. It controls all your vital functions. Forgive yourself and everyone else before you go to sleep, and healing will take place much more rapidly.

—Joseph Murphy

Self-Sabotage

Jorge was a 43-year-old lawyer who was sent to our clinic by his primary care physician to see our cardiologist. He had been diagnosed with elevated cholesterol and borderline hypertension (elevated blood pressure). Jorge complained of increased anxiety and not being able to sleep well. The doctor wanted him to lose at least forty pounds, or he would have to start him on medication. My partner, Dr. Schnur, gave him the option and Jorge chose our EliteFitForever program instead of the meds.

Jorge lived a very high-stress life. On a stress scale of one to ten, he stated he was an eleven. Jorge traveled at least ten days per month on business and had many late business dinners along with a very full social calendar. Jorge's biggest challenge was he did not take time to take care of himself. When it came to diet, he would often skip meals or grab something on the run. The last time he was on any type of exercise regimen was when he was in college, twenty-plus years ago. Like most successful professionals I work with, Jorge's focal point was career, not health.

To create a real program of stress management and eventually Stress Mastery, we must balance the Five Life Categories.

1. Career
2. Finance

3. Health
4. Relationships
5. Spiritual/Self-Improvement

Jorge's focus changed drastically with his visit to our clinic. His motivation stemmed from the simple fact that he was scared to death. Jorge's father had died at the age of fifty from a massive heart attack. Jorge's high stress lifestyle coupled with his elevated blood pressure and cholesterol, and his sharp decrease in energy levels, was a serious wake-up call. I did not have to convince him that he needed to change his lifestyle; he was willing and ready to get started.

Jorge's first thirty days in his program were amazing; he dropped 18 pounds on the scale, and actually lost 21 pounds of fat while gaining three pounds of muscle. Dr. Schnur was equally encouraged as Jorge's blood pressure dropped to an optimal range and his cholesterol fell 65 points. Jorge was thrilled; he loved his new lifestyle and his new look. He was wearing a size of clothing he had not worn in years and looked ten years younger. He did not have any problems following his program even while traveling on business as it was tailored to his needs and particular lifestyle.

Jorge continued to make fabulous progress for the next couple of months. In as little as ten weeks, Jorge dropped 30 pounds of fat and gained eight pounds of muscle. His waist dropped seven inches; his health, along with his energy levels, was the best it had been in twenty years. At this point, everything would begin to change. This is when Jorge informed Alex, his dietician, that he was going to take a short break. He said he would take a couple of weeks off, and then he would return. I tried calling him myself and with all my might attempted to talk him out of this, but he was persistent.

Those two weeks turned into six months. When Jorge finally returned to see Dr. Schnur, his doctor, he had gained all the weight back and an extra ten pounds. Jorge had left Dr. Schnur with no choice but to start him on medication to control his blood pressure and cholesterol. Jorge felt embarrassed when we sat in my office to talk. He could not explain what had happened; he basically just fell apart and went right back to his old habits. I surprised him with my reply. I told him, "What happened to you is normal. It's not your fault!"

What happened to Jorge is common of every client I work with if they let their guard down and don't follow the plan. Jorge had changed his entire life only to snap back to his old habits and life patterns. To change we must understand the intricate working of our mind. Anytime we try to change a behavior or habit, we have to go through a certain process. It does not matter what you want to change; there is a distinct process that must happen before it becomes part of you. When we change our life we assume a new role. That role might be an ex-smoker, healthy dieter, exercise persona or even new spiritual beliefs. The challenge to making a change is this: every new role requires a new self-image or, in other words, a new picture and programs in our mind. Developing that new picture takes time.

The process of creating picture of success involves conquering what I call *Comfort Zone Testing Periods.* I discovered these testing periods in the mid-nineties. During my entire career I have been obsessed with collecting data. When I opened my first personal training center, I would have the trainers keep track of each training session by having the clients sign a dated sheet that was kept in my office. These sheets were color coded so I could tell if a client canceled, didn't show up for their session, or stopped coming in altogether. I would review these sheets with each trainer on a weekly basis to find out the status of every single client at the center.

What I noticed was absolutely astounding. Each client would fall off their program at a certain point of their training, without exception. They would either force themselves to continue or make excuses to stop. During each of the testing periods, clients would cancel, get sick, or quit altogether and if they came in they would be uncharacteristically moody and complaining.

What happened to Jorge, basically, was that he did not pass a Comfort Zone Testing Period that is essential in creating a new habit or behavior. Our habits and behaviors are programmed in our mind. If you change that programming, the picture you have of yourself will then change your life. Jorge knew that in order to keep his weight off and blood pressure down, he would have to maintain a healthy lifestyle.

It truly doesn't matter what we know. What matters is what is programmed in our mind. This changes when we take daily positive action to reset these programs.

We must literally program the habits and behaviors that we want and that is done by overcoming procrastination and doing the work. In the beginning you must create a life of consistency taking action each day to do your work.

To create a balanced life, we must have balance in all of the Five Life Categories. If we have a huge career but we cannot walk across the room without running out of breath, then we are not a success. Likewise, if we have six-pack abs, but cannot pay our bills we are not a success. So what do I mean by doing your work? I mean you must give up excuses and take action. If we are trying to lose weight and get healthy we must follow the right diet and exercise program; *we must do our work*. If we are trying to get out of debt and save money, we must budget; *we must do our work*. If we are looking to build a strong relationship, we must learn to communicate; *we must do our work*. In other words, to change anything in life requires taking action and doing our work. We accomplish this automatically once we understand and overcome procrastination.

Americans are consumed by the quest to find themselves—to find an elusive, omnipresent state of happiness. Most people I meet believe that if they can finally lose their weight, they will then find true happiness. If they find the right mate, they will find happiness. If they win the lottery they will find happiness. In this desperate pursuit of happiness, they will turn to one of the many self-proclaimed self-help gurus of the day.

We are all trying in a desperate way to improve the way we feel about ourselves, to be in control of our financial situation, our children's future, and so many other things. We tend to believe that if only we had a tight grip and control of everything and everyone around us, well, we probably would be happier. Advertisers and late night infomercials prey on this need we have to be more than what we are.

As a nation, we spend millions of dollars buying "self-help" at bookstores and online. We attend seminars, listen to CDs, read books, and watch television shows. All of these aids can be helpful, but they don't represent the solution we are all seeking.

In order to achieve the goals we are striving for, we have to change our habits from the core.

To change these programmed habits, we must take consistent action until the so-called action becomes automatic. I have never met anyone who did not want to change at least something about themselves; they all seem to be waiting for that magic moment to start. *Procrastination*, resistance to change, leads us to a life of excuses and regrets. I will reveal the answer to scientifically overcoming procrastination and creating the life you want by balancing the Five Life Categories. I also give you a dozen techniques that will keep you moving forward when confronted with *procrastination*.

The Power of the Mind

The mind is very complex and powerful, but we can learn to tap into its abundant energy. In order to be successful, we have to create a balance between a healthy body and a healthy mind. How we take care of our health will determine whether we take action or succumb to the procrastination trap of many tomorrows. In fact, once you truly understand how your mind works, you will be able to make life's hard times easier and life's good times even greater and be able to take complete control of your body and health.

Many people do not realize that our brain controls our body's reactions. We are born with a brain that is much more complex than most advanced computers. Scientists claim that people use less than ten percent of their brain's capabilities. Can you imagine what could be possible if we doubled its output to twenty percent?

Our brain contains as many as 100 billion cells and has the ability to process up to 100 million bits of information per hour. Our brain weighs only 2-3% of our body weight but uses 20-30% of the body's oxygen and glucose. It takes care of all our bodily functions and is responsible for balancing billions of cells through the autonomic nervous system. *This system also determines how much self-control you will have at any given moment.* What I find truly amazing is that every thought we have actually has an effect on how our brain functions, which translates to our body functions, which includes everything from our energy levels to our digestion to memory.

Dr. John Hagelin, a quantum physicist, made a great statement: ***"Our body is really the product of our thoughts."*** This observation is so powerful when it comes to any type of program to change our body and health. The fact is our thoughts have a profound effect on the *stress response* and it's this effect that determines whether we do our work or put it off for tomorrow. Procrastination and action are controlled by the state of the body's chemistry at any given time. The thought affects the brain, which becomes the chemist for our body and this creates the chemistry in our environment or our body. It's this chemistry that drives us to respond or to react. In other words, self-discipline can actually be broken down to a relatable science.

My first real experience with the power of the mind was when I found the book *The Power of Positive Thinking* by Norman Vincent Peale. It was the first time I took control of my life by controlling my thoughts. Ever since I read that book, I have dedicated a great part of my time to working and studying how the mind not only affects our body but how it affects all of our life categories.

When I became aware of how the mind can work for or against you, I began mastering techniques to tap the enormous power. These techniques became The Ten Success Principles that I teach in my coaching practice, in my *Stress Mastery Course* and in the new book, *The Seven Steps to Stress Mastery*.

One of the techniques I use in coaching is the power of visualization. I picked this up during my bodybuilding days from Arnold Schwarzenegger. Arnold would talk about how he would visualize exactly how he would look for each competition. I followed his advice to the letter. I would cut out pictures of the exact physique I wanted and then paste a picture of my face onto the body. I would practice thirty minutes each night, visualizing my perfect body. I might have been born with bad genetics, but I trained my mind to help me to become a champion bodybuilder. I changed my body, my metabolism, and my attitude by understanding the power of the mind. I went from being one of the fattest kids in school to a bodybuilding champion.

I have studied the influence of the mind on the body through psychology courses, brain science, prosperity teachings; I have studied books, seminars, tapes, coaches and role models. Most importantly, I have lived these techniques and principles in my own life. Truth be told, since I have learned how to take control of my mind, I have never failed to reach my goals and have never felt out of balance. When I help a client truly grasp the power that they really do possess as an individual, they never fail to reach their goals—never. Once you begin to understand the science of self-discipline, you then have the ability to set your life course and overcome procrastination.

I had many destructive habits (that I thought were normal) built into my life, only to discover that I had been programmed to have them involuntarily. We all have the potential to tap into our mind's unlimited resources; but first, we *must understand* how the mind works and why we sabotage our best efforts.

The Components of Your Mind

There are three components that make up the mind. They are as follows:

1. Conscious mind
2. Subconscious mind
3. Superconscious mind

Each of these three parts of the mind has a profound effect on the actions we take and the results that we receive.

The Conscious Mind: The Captain

Our conscious mind identifies incoming information. This information is received from our senses: sight, sound, smell, taste, and touch. Our conscious mind is the analytical part of the mind. It helps us to reason. It also serves as our center of logical thinking and gives us the power of dissertation. The major functions of the conscious mind involve learning and helping us to be realistic. The conscious mind is the boss, many times referred to as the CEO of the mind.

It is the conscious part of the mind that gives us the power to directly change our lives. When the conscious mind is turned on we are responsive and directed to taking positive action. Since the conscious mind is capable of holding only one thought at a time we are in control of the data input. This data is computed directly into our subconscious mind to create a desired action.

Our conscious mind works like a captain of a submarine. The captain sees everything that is going on through the submarine's periscope and then relays the information to the crew (subconscious mind); it's the crew that is steering the submarine, not the captain. The captain is the conscious mind giving orders to the action-oriented subconscious mind. The conscious mind also is the key to mindfulness training because it allows us to focus on one thing and shuts down the chatter of the subconscious mind. The conscious mind is located in the prefrontal cortex of the brain. It is this area of the brain that brings on responsive actions of change along with optimal well-being and health.

The Subconscious Mind: The Crew

In many ways the subconscious mind is much like the disk storage on a computer. It is used to store the programs and data that the computer needs to operate with. Your conscious mind is like the processor on the computer, which retrieves the programs and data and processes them to operate your body.

An example of how the subconscious mind works is when we are driving a car long distance and become 'lost in our thoughts' only to find we are miles down the road without any conscious recall of the intervening countryside through which we have traveled. Our subconscious mind carried on, allowing us to drive the car quite successfully during this period. Another time might be when we 'unconsciously' turn in the direction towards our workplace on our day off, when we 'consciously' wanted to go somewhere else. All these unconscious programs are of great benefit most of the time as they automatically help us to conduct our lives, leaving our conscious mind free to explore all of the new thoughts. Unfortunately, there are some unconscious or subconscious programs that are not beneficial to us and they can strongly work against us. It's these programs, beliefs and habits that cause us to procrastinate and hold us back from creating the life we want.

It is important to understand how our values, beliefs and habits were programmed. During the first seven years of our life the brain operates at a theta wave length, which is basically a hypnotic state. The subconscious mind is like an MP3 player straight out of the box. The first seven years of life it records everything in its environment and we begin to learn how to live in this world and fit into our tribe. It really does not matter what we tell our children, it only matters what actions we take.

The subconscious is also where our autonomic nervous system resides and controls our bodily functions. In this system we have our survival responses that basically determine if we take action or procrastinate. I will go into more detail on this later.

Let's take another look at our submarine. If the conscious mind were the captain of the submarine, the subconscious would be its crew. The captain (conscious mind) of the submarine peers through the periscope and relays the orders to turn right or left. The crew (subconscious mind) receives the orders and makes the turn. The crew (subconscious mind) has no idea if they are heading straight for an iceberg or to the open seas, they cannot see where they are going; they just do what they are told. But it's the crew (subconscious mind) that is taking the action, not the captain (conscious mind). On the other hand, the crew may put the submarine on automatic pilot (habits, beliefs, and values) and let it guide itself. Many of us live on automatic pilot. It is said we have 60,000 thoughts a day. That is a lot of orders going into our subconscious! The problem is that it's usually the same thoughts over and over again.

The subconscious mind does not think or reason; it reacts. Our subconscious reacts to whatever it is programmed for through our conscious mind. If the input is positive, then the action will be positive. If the input is negative, then the action will be negative. What we must understand is that this input comes from everything and everybody around us, and it will affect every aspect of our lives from our career, finances, health, relationships and even our spiritual development.

Change Your Thoughts, Change Your Life

Managing the subconscious mind is key to all your success and failure. You begin to control your subconscious by managing your thoughts and your conscious input. When we change our programming, our thoughts automatically become productive and everything changes including our health. Here are some valuable points on the subconscious mind:

1. The subconscious mind accepts whatever your conscious mind sends it; the subconscious will not argue with you.
2. If your thoughts are good, your subconscious will project good.
3. You have the power to choose your conscious thoughts. It is your choice what to feed your subconscious. Choose health and happiness, and that is what you will receive.
4. Whatever statements you choose to say are directly loaded into your subconscious. It is essential to be accountable for everything you say. I will fail, I can't lose weight, I have a slow metabolism—these are orders from the captain, you!
5. Your subconscious has no sense of humor—it cannot take a joke. It believes everything you tell it. "I'm too old to get in shape." "At my age, you just start breaking down." "I look at the cake and gain ten pounds."
6. The subconscious is always about what you choose. You are the captain of your subconscious. Choose health, choose success, choose love, and choose happiness!
7. Subconscious programs control our unconscious actions or habits.
8. The subconscious connects us to the superconscious mind and our higher power.
9. Subconscious controls our overall health.
10. The most powerful statements to the subconscious mind are "I AM…" These statements can be empowering or disempowering.

Now that you are starting to understand how the mind works, it would seem simple to make any changes we want in our lives. If you are the captain, all you have to do is give the orders to the crew—to lose weight, quit smoking, stop being late or change any bad habit you may have. We all know it's not that simple. We have to monitor our conscious thoughts, and we have to reprogram our subconscious beliefs and values to create new habits. Simple does not always mean easy. *Changing the subconscious takes work along with consistent action.*

The New Year's Resolution Phenomenon

Every year, that magic date will come around on the calendar—January first. This is the date when we all decide to finally change our lives. We promise ourselves that we will lose weight, we will find the right relationship, make more money, change jobs, write a book; the list is endless. Unfortunately, most of us never succeed in carrying out our goals.

It has nothing to do with determination, and it has everything to do with programming and our ability to conquer procrastination.

You will easily know if you are stuck in subconscious programming by taking a look at your life and your goals. If January every year you have the same goals from the previous year to lose weight, stop smoking, change jobs, etc., there is a pretty good chance you are stuck. To accomplish any type of change, you have to become the programmer of your life. To create the new programs, you must be able to take consistent action. In other words, you have to activate your *self-discipline mechanism* and do the work that is needed to get the result. For any type of long-term results, we must program new habits. To create new subconscious habits, we must do the work on a consistent basis.

Habits

All habits, both good and bad, have been programmed in your computer (subconscious). Unfortunately, much of it is without your consent. Whatever is programmed determines the action you will take on a regular basis; in other words, your habits. Your subconscious has been receiving information since the day you were born; it records every single moment of your life. The first seven years of life our brain and subconscious operates in a hypnotic state.

Our first programmers are our parents who pass on their beliefs and values to us by raising us and instilling their personal, cultural, and other value systems. If your household was positive, proactive, and was about becoming successful, your programming would be the same. On the other hand, if your household was dysfunctional, full of drama and negativity, you will have those same traits. Most people will follow their family traits unless they understand how to change deeply embedded habits and patterns. These programmed traits have a direct effect on the actions we take and the life we ultimately will build.

There are many other influences on our early programming besides our parents. Other programmers are our teachers, role models, coaches, television, the media, and the culture where we come from, religion, and other value systems. They influence us through individual experiences and peer pressure from childhood to adulthood. Programming from television, radio, magazines, and all the advertisements tell us what to wear, what kind of car to drive, what foods give us pleasure, and even what we are supposed to look like. Many parents use the television as a babysitter and with the brain and subconscious in full recording mode it's no wonder that as adults we cannot get out of our own way.

Imagine the influence of subconscious programming when it comes to weight loss. Just watch the ads that are shown. One will tell us to go to a fast-food restaurant because you deserve a break. The next ad will then tell you to buy a pill to help you finally lose the weight. When the holidays roll around, all the advertisement you see is about having these large meals with all your family gathered at the table. The ads will promote overconsumption of all types of food.

In America, we have been programmed to value the notion that we need more, especially when it comes to food. We spend billions every year to lose weight, but until we understand how the mind works and its direct effect on our self-discipline mechanism, we will ride the diet roller coaster and be setting the same goals on January 1 every year.

On a daily basis we see ads that describe variety products to extend life, improve sex, find the perfect mate, and become rich overnight; it's easy and doesn't require work! These "Get Results Fast" programs prey on our desire to change but offer no real answers. The *TRUTH* is this: In order to change we have to create new habits or programs that support the change we desire.

The Challenge of Changing a Habit

Our subconscious programming is where we hold our habits, beliefs, and values. If we want to change a habit, we must change the programming. *The challenge here is that the subconscious is designed never to change.* Our subconscious is what is called homeostatic. Homeostasis is defined as a condition in which the body's internal environment remains relatively constant; it is not supposed to change. Our subconscious mind controls our body mainly through the autonomic nervous system. The autonomic nervous system is responsible for all the mechanisms and systems needed to keep our bodies alive—the beating of our heart, the blinking of our eyes, the function of our organs, our body temperature, and even determines whether you will or will not do what you're supposed to do, in other words, it determines if you will do your work. This is why our subconscious mind translates its need for homeostasis to the part of the mind that creates action.

We are basically built to survive and the brain uses a lot of fuel so it's wired to conserve energy. By lumping events and things into categories the brain creates a habit to conserve energy leading us to do things automatically. If you take a close look most of us have the same morning routine. We get up, get dressed, drive the same route to work and then we unconsciously do our best to get through the day so we can come home to the same routine we had yesterday.

The subconscious also manages our bodily functions; for example, our body's normal temperature stays approximately at 98.6 degrees. There is not much difference between the number 98.6 and the number 102, right? Not really. When it comes to our body's temperature, this difference represents a significant change. The body's systems go into action to get its temperature back to 98. This involves millions of cells for all this to happen. You don't have to tell your body to get to work; it's on automatic pilot to rebalance your entire system, it's homeostatic.

Another example is when we get stressed out. If we are stressed about being late for an important appointment and we are stuck in traffic our body will respond from the subconscious survival program and kick in the sympathetic nervous systems and the stress response. The body will react and get ready to fight or flight even though we are stuck in a car. This response cannot be shut off—only managed—and the response can't tell the difference if we are stuck in traffic or we are facing down a saber-toothed tiger…it just responds. In today's world there seems to be a lot of saber-toothed tigers.

When it comes to personal development of any kind it is essential to understand that the same process that unconsciously protects our body is standing guard over our habits, both good and bad.

The subconscious mind and its programs are protected against change by what is known as your *comfort zone*. The comfort zone has one purpose—it is designed to make sure you do not change the program of the subconscious mind. The comfort zone is essential for our survival but it is also the saboteur of all change. The comfort zone is the resistance; the fear we feel when we attempt any type of personal development. What is programmed in your comfort zone comes easy for you; it's automatic. Your subconscious does not know smoking is bad for you. You know smoking is bad, but the truth is it doesn't matter what you know; it only matters what is programmed in the subconscious. Most of us go through life and wonder why we do the things we do. We set out with good intentions to change our lives and seem to always end back where we started or even worse off than when we began. We have good intention and start a new task with all the gusto in the world only to have it all come to a screeching halt with *procrastination and self-sabotage creating resistance* to any type of change.

Breaking any habit means we have to confront the resistance and step outside of our comfort zone to create change. Wishing for these changes just is not enough. We do not realize that our surroundings are influencing us every day of our lives. Everything we say and do is either helping us grow or keeping us stuck in a life we wish would change. We need to monitor our conscious mind and only let thoughts and messages into our subconscious that would empower us. We must follow a system that works with our physiology as we work to create a new psychology of change. In *The Seven Steps to Stress Mastery* I have perfected a systematic approach in changing our habits. In this book I will give you a preview of the dozen techniques that work on reprogramming your habits in ten minutes or less by breaking through procrastination and the comfort zone.

Using the Ten Minute Life Plan techniques have only one purpose and that is to drive you outside the comfort zone so you can do the work that needs to be done to create change.

The Superconscious Mind

The song we're composing already exists in potential. Our work is to find it. **—Steven Pressfield**

While the conscious and subconscious aspects of our mind are closely aligned with our physical shell or body, the superconscious mind is super physical. In other words, it exists at a level extending beyond our space-time continuum.

If we looked at our example of a computer, we can liken it to the Internet, which enables us to connect to every other computer in the world, and the people using those computers. But with the superconscious connection we do not need any other technology than what we are born with. Through the superconscious it is possible for us to connect to every other mind on the planet. However, connecting to our superconscious opens up much wider doorways than just linking to other minds. It is also that aspect of our being that exists before we were born and survives our death. Some also call this aspect the higher self.

Your belief system might be along the lines of atheism or agnosticism as you perceive it on a conscious level. You may or may not believe that there is an aspect of your *being* that extends beyond your birth and death. But the truth of the matter is that your subconscious and superconscious care very little about what your conscious mind believes; they continue influencing your life as best they can. While you ignore that 'small voice within' on many an occasion, you almost always find that it is to your detriment.

Roles the Superconscious Performs: Our Life Plan

It is our superconscious mind that holds the blueprint or script for all that we have set out to achieve in our current lifetime. Imagine if we could tap into this plan and discover why we have chosen to experience all the pain and joys of our life experience? How much more effective could we be if we really understood what our real life plan is?

You may consciously believe that you have no underlying plan in your life. However, if you reviewed your life closely you will find in your life 'certain things happened' (you may call them chance or coincidence), which helped or forced you to change directions in ways that were ultimately beneficial to you. Wouldn't it be great to become more aware of the signals that we are getting from our superconscious? This could help us to smooth the transitions brought on by those 'life corrections' we all seem to face at certain times of our lives

In my past work I have been instructed by many so-called experts not to mention or talk about God. They believed it would hurt me in the corporate arena and may turn some people off. I don't know if this is right or not but as I have gotten more established I have decided that I need to be true to myself. I believe in God and it is with God's grace that I have lived such a blessed life. During the good and the bad times, I have had one constant—and that is God.

The superconscious mind works as the connector to God, spirit, higher consciousness, the universe, or the higher self. This is our spiritual self, our connection, our guiding voice, our influence in life that gives us our particular direction, mission and purpose.

The superconscious is our universal connector, our guide to the angels and spirit guides that give us divine intuition and insight. I personally am a big believer in connecting to the superconscious before I write or give a lecture. I will say The Lord's Prayer and meditate until I am in a state of Zen before I speak or write. This ritual may take all of five minutes but it is essential for me because it connects me to a higher power.

If I feel blocked I will do an Emotional Freedom Technique (EFT), also called Tapping. If I feel stressed I will exercise to release any tightness in my body. I do these mini-rituals because they connect me and shut off my chattering mind, which creates higher focus. When I am connected I find the message is flawless.

I always say, "I don't believe in theory; I believe in science." But, I also believe in miracles and I am careful not to label events as good or bad. I believe that we are all here to express our higher purpose and to live our best life and I present this work and all I have ever accomplished as a work from some place way beyond myself. The superconscious mind is the connector to the Divine Intelligence and the answer to life's most pressing questions and most incredible discoveries. God will guide you if you trust and listen. As I write this I am reading one of my first and greatest teacher's new books *I Can See Clearly Now* by Dr. Wayne Dyer. In the book Dr. Dyer chronicles his life and discusses how there were no accidents, and that every event had one purpose and that was to guide his mission through this lifetime.

The superconscious is accessed through our subconscious mind. That is why it is essential we captain our ship with good conscious thoughts, especially the words we speak. When we are connected it's that exciting feeling you get when you have a new idea or when you're working on a project that you truly love. It is when everything that you are doing seems to work effortlessly. It is the source of all pure creativity and has access to all stored information, past and present. People, information, ideas, problem solving, all comes naturally.

This is when everything in your life is at a balanced pace and everything just seems to work. To achieve this state, we must watch our input into the subconscious because if the input is consistently negative it will keep us in a lower state of consciousness. In this lower state we experience depression and illness and more importantly, we cannot access the higher state thus causing us to live a life of lack.

There are examples of people who live their lives from this special place all around us. Watching Oprah skillfully interviewing a guest, Tiger Woods making an incredible golf shot, Joel Osteen giving a service from the heart. You can see they are connected.

When you study people like Dr. Wayne Dyer, Albert Einstein, Thomas Edison, Bill Gates, Nelson Mandela, Henry Ford, Mother Teresa, Jesus Christ, and Buddha, you see they lived life on another level. The author Napoleon Hill referred to this power as infinite intelligence. In his incredible book *Think and Grow Rich,* he states that our superconscious is the universal storehouse of knowledge. He states that when you have a pressing problem, just tap into this infinite intelligence and you will not only receive the answer, but you will always receive the correct answer. Napoleon Hill also states that all great success enjoyed by hundreds of wealthy men and women he interviewed over the years were achieved as a direct result of this tapping into infinite intelligence or the superconscious mind.

Getting the Power

The purpose of this book is not to convert you into being a spiritual person, but to give you the tools and understanding that it takes to build a life that is of your making by taking action on a daily basis and by overcoming procrastination. In other words, the tools in this book are designed for you to take action—to do the work. It is important to understand that there are guides and forces that science cannot explain, but also cannot ignore. From everything Gandhi accomplished to what Steve Jobs created to Thomas Edison inventing the light bulb—it's a power that is very real. It is a power that will change you and your life forever.

Every day, I personally tap into this power. I feel it when I'm training and lifting weights (that are supposed to be impossible for my age). I feel it when I am with a client. My work flows effortlessly, as it is while I am writing this chapter. Many times when I see a client I instinctively know what the person needs. Whether it's a kind word or strong motivation, I allow myself to follow my gut, and it's never wrong. When I give a seminar, I never script myself; I always know from the energy of the crowd which way to focus the talk. Everything I do, when tapping into this force, seems effortless and sheer pleasure. *The Ten Minute Life Plan* techniques are designed to help you to connect to this state.

What is the key to tap into this power on a regular basis? It is the same key that I teach in my *Livin' In The Green Zone* coaching courses and in my books, *The NEW Stress-Response Diet and Lifestyle Program* and *TRUTH.* The key is to activate our self-control mechanism. It's about managing our survival responses and having a distinct reason or purpose to change. I defined my career mission back in 1985 while working in a Family Practice Clinic. I wanted to motivate, educate, and inspire people to live their best life. How does this work in my life? Well, first, let's take the **motivation** part of my mission. I am a coach, I will always push you to live the life you deserve and the life you truly want. I will push you to make the changes that must be made for you to reach your goals. I will encourage you when you are down and high-five you when you win.

Second, I will **educate** you on how to do this. It is not enough to be told to change; you have to understand how to change. Education is the key for anyone to step outside their comfort zone and seek true transformation. You have to understand why you do the things you do and more importantly the reason these changes will work for you. The old saying that knowledge is power is so true.

Third, **inspiration** is about walking the talk. I know what I teach works because the bottom line is I live it every day. If I can keep over one hundred pounds off for over thirty years, anyone can. I also created my career and that even includes my personal job description. In other words, there were no jobs that I wanted to do so I created one and its exact description. I have traveled the world and given lectures on four continents; I have built businesses in three countries and developed my own supplements, exercise videos and published two books. I don't merely *believe* that the Green Zone Productivity System works; I *know* it works because I live it—every day! In *TRUTH* I take personal development to another level. Since I turned fifty years old I have had to revamp my personal programs and this is what drove me to write *TRUTH*.

With my mission steadfast it gives me my life's purpose, which is to bring medicine and wellness and fitness together. I have dreamed of medical personnel working side by side with dietitians, life coaches and exercise specialists since I entered the medical field in the early eighties.

In the years of 2010 to 2016, I developed a highly scientific wellness program after testing over 4000 subjects. In these years, I learned that we, as humans, are built for one thing and one thing only: survival. If you master the survival responses that include the body and mind, you will eventually shift your consciousness levels toward living in a state where the outside environment no longer affects your inner being. This is Stress Mastery, and I give you the exact steps to achieve this in *The Seven Steps of Stress Mastery.*

Chapter Two: Resistance to Change

Sometimes we have to step out of our comfort zones. We have to break the rules. And we have to discover the sensuality of fear. We need to face it, challenge it, dance with it.   — Kyra Davis

The Comfort Zone

Many people have heard the term *comfort zone* but do not fully understand its full impact on our lives. The comfort zone protects your subconscious programming. The subconscious mind's programs are the actions that you are comfortable performing, right or wrong; they are your unconscious habits, beliefs, and values. For instance, we get up in the morning and brush our teeth. We do not even think about it or question it; we just do it. Brushing our teeth is part of our comfort zone. If you have ever forgotten your toothbrush on a trip and couldn't brush your teeth, you know how uncomfortable that can make you feel. That's how our comfort zone works.

It is essential to understand that the comfort zone protects the subconscious programs. These programs are your habits, and values. Well, I should say they are really seeds that were planted when you were a child. You will recall from Chapter One that during the first seven years of life our brain operates on what is called a theta brainwave level. Theta level is basically hypnotic; in other words, the brain is working in a state of hypnosis and recording everything that happens in our surroundings. Our first programs, our first beliefs, our first values were seeds planted from outside environment. It's these seeds that create resistance, procrastination and many of our life frustrations, especially if you are trying to grow and improve.

When it comes to diet, exercise, health, personal development, money, spiritual development, career growth or relationships, there are many comfort zone 'programs' in our mind of which we must be aware.

Here are a few:

- Eating fat will make me fat.
- It's normal to get aches and pains as we age.
- Exercise is about "no pain, no gain."
- If I expect good things I will get the opposite, so I expect the worse so I don't get disappointed.
- Vitamins will make me fat.
- God will punish me.
- I'm too old to go back to school.
- I am one person; I can't make a difference.
- I should lose the weight first, and then start exercising.
- As we age, energy levels drop.
- I'm addicted to chocolate.
- I will start tomorrow.
- Money doesn't grow on trees
- I can't write a book; no one would want it.
- I love carbohydrates.
- The rich get richer and the poor get poorer.
- Don't trust anyone!
- People don't change.
- I should act my age.
- I have a slow metabolism.
- You can't teach an old dog new tricks.
- Social Media is for the young; I'm too old.
- I have bad genetics.
- Technology is ruining the world.
- The younger generation is lazy.

These programs are designed to keep you where you are at in life. *The moment you decide to change all hell breaks loose within your mind.* When this happens we experience *resistance* and we have one of two things happen: We will either put off starting something that will improve our life, or we start and out of nowhere we sabotage our efforts.

If you have ever watched the television series Mad Men you will see how the lead character, Don Draper, gears every ad toward emotion. Emotion can link a product or action to the subconscious. Once the link is there you take action and buy the product. Because such emotion is attached you will find yourself defending the action or purchase. In the 1950s smoking was marketed as glamorous although in reality it makes us smell, stains our teeth and it kills us. Yet, if you didn't smoke you weren't in the hip club. Beer ads, fast food ads, medication ads, must-have clothing ads, new diets, anti-aging and miracle skin care, lose weight easy and fast, become rich overnight—the list is endless and marketing geniuses know just how to get that message to provoke emotion which causes you to take action.

Change in life takes work and consistent action. I understand that this can be hard especially when you deserve a break today at McDonald's. *TRUTH* and *The Ten Minute Life Plan* will give you the tools and answers to create change. Change comes when we step outside the comfort zone of our life.

Comfort Zone and Resistance to Change

Are you paralyzed with fear? That's a good sign. Fear is good. Like self-doubt, fear is an indicator. Fear tells us what we have to do. Remember one rule of thumb: the more scared we are of a work or calling, the more sure we can be that we have to do it.

—Steven Pressfield

In my thirty plus years in the personal development field I have read hundreds of books, taken countless courses and have had teachers from all walks of life. But, if I had to pick just one book, one teacher that changed my life forever, it would be Steven Pressfield. Steven Pressfield is an incredible writer of inspirational fiction. His book, that later became a movie starring Matt Damon and Will Smith, *The Legend of Bagger Vance,* ranks as my favorite and most inspirational movie of all time. I could relate to the movie about a war hero who had a traumatic experience in the war and upon his return took to drinking and just getting by in life. Before the war he had been an incredible golfer and was the town's golden boy. As it turns out our hero is put into a situation that the town needs him to play a match game against two golf legends. Our hero can no longer play the game he had mastered early in life and sure enough, out of nowhere, Bagger Vance, a golf caddie (who really is an angel) shows up in the middle of the night to help our hero. The entire theme of the book and movie is about finding your authentic swing. The swing translated to mean finding and living your true purpose. (Side note: the book is even better than the movie as the Bagger Vance character is really magnified but the movie is spectacular.)

I have watched this movie hundreds of times and each time I breakdown and cry. I related to the movie because my grandfather, who taught me the game of golf, raised me as a child and it was something that we shared dearly. More than that, the movie stirs something so deep within me that I actually shake. It wasn't this book that changed my life—it was Pressfield's nonfiction work *The War of Art* that transformed my work ethic and my entire life right along with it. In *The War of Art*, Pressfield talks about what holds people back from living their dream lives. He aims the books toward artist such as writers and painters but he explains that any dream not realized, any type of health regimen, any personal development, any spiritual calling and any entrepreneurial venture or further education of any type is affected by a force. What is this force? It is *resistance—the comfort zone in action.*

I have been lecturing and writing on personal development since the early nineties. I have understood the mind and how we have to program in life exactly what we want. When Rhonda Byrne wrote the book *The Secret* I had already been living those principles for years. It was not until I read *The War of Art* that I really got off my ass and started realizing my potential. What was the secret? I did my work! Yes, Pressfield's message is simple: you have to become a pro and just do your work. No excuses, no sick days, no snow days, no holidays, it was all about doing what you need to do to create the life you want, it's about doing your work.

Resistance is the comfort zone telling you to start tomorrow or you're too busy or you're not good enough; its tools are procrastination and fear. The comfort zone isn't this nice little fuzzy place that makes you a little uncomfortable when you want to change. No, the comfort zone is evil. It is what holds us back and causes us to live a life unrealized. Pressfield calls this resistance "the force that you feel when you know you should do something but decide you will do it later," and as we know, later never comes. ***Success comes from action but resistance will kick you in the gut to stop that action at all costs.***

My experience with the comfort zone and its resistance was interesting because there are parts of my life when I kick resistance's butt, and there are parts where resistance brings me to my knees. When it comes to diet and exercise, 99% of people struggle—but not me. I never (or very rarely) miss a workout and I have maintained that consistency for over thirty years. My secret formula is this: when the alarm goes off in the morning, if my feet hit the floor, I train! Now understand that I work out at 3:30a.m., so I am tired many times when the bell sounds. But this simple system continues to work for me. I have also programmed my lifestyle system within my own comfort zone so it becomes automatic.

Comfort zone programming and resistance seem to challenge me more in my career as I want to grow, expand and venture into uncharted territories in wellness and personal development. I came from a blue collar family whose philosophy was to fit in to the system and avoid ruffling feathers; but in my lifetime I have created many firsts. I opened the first personal training studio in Miami, Florida. I was one of the first in the United States to work with wellness programs for 70, 80 and 90 year olds. I opened the first active adult training centers. I was the first to bring wellness to the country of Panama creating an entire new industry. I was the first to put together the testing for the Stress-Response. I opened the first medical-wellness clinics. I have also authored three books, done infomercials and lectured around the world.

I can tell you only this fact: With each new project I was scared shitless because of dozens of factors created by resistance and the need for my comfort zone to corral me.

Action Is the Answer

What is the *Livin' In The Green Zone* course? It is a program for learning the techniques of taking action and overcoming our fears. *It's about living in the Green Zone of our nervous system which gives us the ability to respond to life instead of reacting to it* (more on this in Chapter Four, Procrastination; I Will Start Tomorrow). It's about doing the things that you are supposed to do when you are supposed to do them. It's about ending procrastination and increasing performance. You cannot see the comfort zone but you sure can feel it when you step outside of it. It's that feeling that you're not good enough. It's the questions that pop into your head. What if I fail? What if no one buys? What if I end up bankrupt? What if, what if, what if…?

Here is the great news: When you finally make that decision and start toward your goals and begin to take action you begin to tap into the superconscious mind. When this happens the universal energies, the angels, God, start to bring you a flood of ideas. The right people, the right circumstances seem to magically appear. Everything you need to do your life's work and realize your dreams begin to fall into place. When you confront the comfort zone and the resistance you begin to grow in ways that you just cannot explain. *The Ten Minute Life Plan* techniques are geared to help you switch on this incredible power of action.

People ask me if as we get older if it gets easier to confront our comfort zone resistance or our fears. My answer is NO. It does not get easier. Every day you have to take action and make decisions that will empower you.

If you go on a diet and lose weight, you can't hit your goal then return to the same habits that made you fat to start with. This goes for any type of growth, personal development or spiritual advancement. Each day you have to take action if you want to maintain and keep moving forward. Life is all about challenging us to live our best virtues and challenging us to grow past our shortcomings. I can say this though, once you understand the art of taking action you will no longer participate in self-sabotaging actions. It is all about living within in a system. I teach more about this in the *Livin' In The Green Zone* course which is a step-by-step system to help you to step up against comfort zone resistance.

Redesigning Your Comfort Zone

Action is the key to change and what we have programmed in our subconscious mind determines the actions that we take on a regular basis.

Let's take a step back and look at the early programmers of our subconscious mind. Many of our early programmers were merely passing to us their own programs. Many of our beliefs, values and habits are passed down from generation to generation. Good intentioned parents try to protect us from the pain of failing, while our schools work to conform our way of learning and our spiritual guidance is one of teaching us to fear the wrath of God.

These teachings become deep unconscious programs that are protected by the resistance of the comfort zone. In the comfort zone, most of the unconscious programming we have been exposed to is not necessarily geared toward our growth and when we set out to create a new lifestyle or new habits, we have to be willing to step outside our comfort zone and be uncomfortable with its resistance. Stepping out is simply doing the work and taking action. It's all about following a plan.

The very first step, we must be willing to change. In *Livin' In The Green Zone* the number one Success Principle is *Purpose*. In order for you to tackle the comfort zone and all its power of resistance you must have a strong WHY!

Change does not come from common sense; it comes from a strong want and purpose.

This may sound a little silly, but after working with thousands of clients, you would not believe what they would do to protect their comfort zones. I have seen clients who have had heart attacks and have pacemakers who would rather die than give up smoking. I have seen diabetics who refuse to manage their disease even after losing a foot. It does not matter how much the doctor preaches to patients to take care of themselves, they just cannot, or should I say will not, modify their lifestyle habits. They succumb to comfort zone resistance and procrastinate on taking action or sabotage their efforts once they do get started.

Much of this reluctance to change is directly related to stress in two ways. First, most of our early programming was given to us during times of stress. Parenting is super stressful in today's fast paced world where both parents work while trying to juggle a job and an infant. The best babysitter for young stressed out parents many times falls to the television. Hours of entertainment and programming that are designed to create a future consumer. You cannot blame the poor stressed out parents who just wanted to steal a moment to catch their breath; yes, more programming as the parents feel a need to escape. If you hurt yourself, your mother would give you a cookie or a comfort food. If you had a bad day at school, you would probably get ice cream. During a stressful period, we automatically turn to the programs of comfort, and our mind doesn't know if the comfort program is healthy or unhealthy.

The second way stress and the stress response sabotages change is it causes us to be in a reactive state and not take the action that we need to take to create change. The stress response fires the sympathetic nervous system for us to react in fight-or-flight mode. When this happens the brain shuts down the self-control mechanism. I will get more into this in the next chapter which I titled Our Survival Responses.

In order to make real change happen, we have to get leverage on ourselves. We have to be willing to face our fears of the comfort zone resistance and do the work needed to create the change we seek. The fear of not having dessert, of going through a holiday and not eating everything on the plate, or fear of having to exercise in front of other people or getting sore muscles, the fear of failing or looking foolish, the fear of rejection, the fear of success—these are all fears, tools of the comfort zone that are designed to prevent you from taking action. We must face these fears to find optimal health, success and peace.

The Comfort Zone Reset

While working in the health and personal development field I have discovered some very interesting characteristics that develop in each one of my clients as they go through their personal development. Whether it's losing weight or changing careers there is a distinct pattern that occurs. These were patterns of some sort of self-sabotage that most times did not make any common sense. I discovered that over a one-year period, there would be four times in which the client would be challenged while creating their new lifestyle. I called these times their *Comfort Zone Testing Periods.*

The testing periods were times when my clients would sabotage themselves for no apparent reason, much like Jorge in the story at the beginning of this book. I discovered that these are the periods where the homeostatic subconscious mind wanted to return to its original programming. In other words, your habits would return to the original comfort zone. This pull is very unconscious and part of the way our mind operates; it can take control of your life. share with you in this audio book. minute sion.   is very powerful indeed.

Most of us go through life and wonder why we do the things we do. We set out with good intentions to change our lives and we always seem to end back where we started or even worse off than where we began. The reason this happens is because to create change we must create new habits. Lasting change only comes when we do the things that need to be done on a daily basis (take action), whether we feel like it or not.

Anyone can lose weight but to lose weight and keep it off is another story. The reason is the comfort zone protects the subconscious. Habits, whether they are so called good habits or bad habits, the subconscious doesn't know the difference. The subconscious reacts to its programs, period!

The Snap Back Effect

One of the early pioneers in self-image psychology was Dr. Maxwell Maltz. In his book *Psycho-Cybernetics*, Dr. Maltz gives his explanation of 'The Snap Back Effect.' He compares our self-image to a rubber band. When it is in its normal shape and size, it represents our current self-image. However, when you put the rubber band between your thumb and index finger and stretch it as far as you can, you are stretching the band beyond its normal limits. He likens this to when we try to perform beyond our current self-image through new routines and behaviors. What happens to the rubber band after a short time is that it 'snaps back' to its original size because it cannot sustain the new position. Stretched beyond its capacity, it will always snap back. So too, when we perform at levels above our current self-image, we cannot sustain the new behaviors because they are inconsistent with the picture we have of ourselves. Our self-image snaps us back to our old behaviors. I read Dr. Maltz's book when I lost the 100 pounds of weight. It was this book and his work that led me from being one of the fattest kids in school to winning seven bodybuilding titles. I had lost 100 pounds three times before and had always gained it back. It wasn't until I understood the concept of changing my self-image.

The Snap Back Effect is when we begin to self-sabotage our efforts to grow. That is why it's important to understand that we all behave according to a picture or portrait that we created about ourselves called our self-image. I break the self-image into three parts: Self-Beliefs, Self-Worth and Self-Esteem.

The comfort zone and all its power of resistance is the protector of the programmed subconscious habits. These programmed habits are designed to remain the same, as the subconscious does not know the difference between a good or bad habit. This state of homeostasis is what causes many to fail in any type of personal development, which includes everything from weight loss to relationships to spiritual advancement. This form of self-sabotage is the Snap Back Effect. Whatever is programmed in your subconscious mind is going to be your end result. Let us take a look at how this effect can impact your earnings.

Let's say you are a sales person with a small territory. You are doing great and soon you are easily making $5,000 per month. You are comfortable with your territory and the money you're making. The management notices that you have really done well in the small territory so they promote you to a larger more lucrative area. You have earned the reputation of a go-getter.

You're excited about the promotion but are feeling a little anxious and uncertain about having a larger territory. You feel pressure, as you believe that everyone is expecting big numbers. Your family is excited about your new promotion and surely you don't want to disappoint them. For some reason you're having trouble making the new area work and you are feeling tired and exhausted to the point you had to see a doctor. Every day you tell yourself, "Tomorrow I will make the calls and be more aggressive," but each day there is another excuse. Your family and friends notice the change because you never seem to feel well. As months go by it becomes apparent to management that you are not cut out for the job. The projected income for a salesperson in that territory is $10-12,000 per month and you are still stuck making $5,000.

Management has lost faith in you and assigns you to a smaller territory, in fact smaller than your original territory and to make matters worse the demographic income of the new territory was $20,000 less per year than your original territory. But, you are not about to be knocked down and with incredible enthusiasm you go to work. You begin to build new sales and work harder than ever. At the end of the month management cannot believe how well you have done for that territory…you've earned $5,000, a record for this area! Plus, you are healthy once again with high energy levels and you even lost ten pounds with this new lease on life.

The above scenario is played out on a regular basis. If you ask any sales manager, they will tell you about this phenomenon. This is the Snap Back Effect in action. Basically, $5,000 is the programmed self-worth of the salesman and no matter how the outside circumstances change he will always snap back. The snap back is the reason lottery winners lose their money within five years and athletes that earn millions of dollars end up broke after their career ends. The same happens when it comes to weight loss. After thirty years in the wellness field, when it comes to losing weight, I know that changing the self-image picture is as important as the diet and exercise program.

New roles in life whether it is your new thinner body, income, new relationships or even new spiritual practices require a new self-image and comfort zone programming.

The Comfort Zone Testing Periods

The body uses pain as a signal to let us know that something may be wrong. When we feel pain in our physical body we will do what's necessary to avoid that pain. For example, if we reach for something and it burns us we will avoid touching it again to avoid that pain. Pain is the tool the body uses to communicate. We are wired to avoid pain thus we pull away or avoid what is causing the pain.

The subconscious mind and comfort zone also uses pain to keep you within your subconsciously programmed habits. The comfort zone resistance is like an electric fence designed to keep you caged in, the moment you get too close it will shock you causing pain or discomfort. The comfort zone uses a powerful tool to protect its programs, habits, values and beliefs. *This tool is fear*. The comfort zone uses fear very wisely. It disguises it as worry, anxiety, jealousy, anger, procrastination, complaining, fear of failure, success, rejection and a host of other phobias that can paralyze us into non-action.

When creating new programs and habits the Snap Back Effect will be ever present and I have found that there are distinct testing periods that we must go through while creating change.

They are as follows:

- **Testing Period One: 30 Days**. It takes thirty days to really start expanding the comfort zone. This 30-day testing period is the hardest because it is when resistance and the comfort zone are the strongest. My coaching program, *Shift Coaching,* is designed to change the programs of the subconscious; thus, shifting your consciousness to a higher level The first Success Principle in *Shift Coaching* is *Purpose*—creating a strong reason to change; creating the WHY. The comfort zone uses all its forces of resistance to stop you so the WHY is important because you are not going to feel like doing the work in the beginning of any type of goal or change.

- **Testing Period Two: 12 weeks**. This testing period occurs after 12 weeks from the point that you started your personal development quest. When it comes to weight loss this is the testing period when many sabotage themselves by undoing everything that worked the months before. This is when our patients hit a plateau and begin to get panicky. In the diet world, this is when the plateau hits. Resistance is super strong at the 12-week mark, as it wants to snap you back to your old programs (habits).

- **Testing Period Three: 6 months.** This is a testing period that really is connected to your self-image. New roles require a new self-image, in other words, as you begin to change you must make sure the picture of your new life match your pictures in your mind, your self-image. I have had clients that have lost over 100 pounds only to lose control and gain it back because people were complimenting them on their weight loss accomplishment. The compliments did not match their self-image, which provoked their stress response programming, and they turned back to eating the comfort foods that they had avoided to lose the weight. The Snap Back Effect is very powerful, and once you're in its grip you have to have the tools to reset your program. In

The Seven Steps to Stress Mastery you are taught the tools as you travel through each step. Each principle is a tool that resets the self-image and controls the Snap Back Effect by creating a new comfort zone for your new role in life. Basically, you are reprogramming the picture you are holding in your mind.

- **Testing Period Four**: **One Year**. When you reach one year from the time you stepped out of your comfort zone and began the personal development quest you then reset your life. It takes one year to create the program of the new habit. When it comes to diet and exercise you now have your program programmed where the comfort zone now can become an ally. If you cheat on your diet or skip a workout you will feel uncomfortable and you will want to stay on track. It does not mean that you can go back to your old habits of eating junk food. It means you *don't* go back to the old habit.

A word of caution is to be very careful when you experience an extremely stressful event because it can trigger the Snap Back Effect. The number of successful clients that fell off the wagon after the attacks on 9/11 shocked me. I could not believe how many clients, who had been successful for 5 or 6 years, suddenly fell completely out of the program and some of them gained back everything they had lost years before. Stress is a deep trigger. A death, divorce, bankruptcy, and even a world event can trigger a snap back.

Chapter Three:
Our Survival Responses

You have power over your mind - not outside events. Realize this, and
you will find strength. — **Marcus Aurelius**

Self-Control Mechanism

Stress Response

In previous publications, I wrote about stress and its effect on our health
and our metabolism. Stress isn't good or bad; it's a response. The stress
response is appropriately called the fight-or-flight stress response and it
is designed to get you out of harm's way without having you overthink
or take time to analyze the situation. The stress response is part of our
survival DNA and is designed to get us to react. You notice any danger
and your body goes into action. The heart pounds, breathing quickens
and the senses go on high alert. These changes in the body are designed
to get you to either fight or flee for your life. Stress hormones flood the
body in a sophisticated way to get the brain and nervous system to make
sure you act quickly and with every ounce of energy you have, without
thought. The stress response was vital to our survival when creatures the
size of high rise-buildings roamed the earth. But in today's world the
body cannot tell the difference between facing a saber-toothed tiger or if
you're running late for an important meeting—it just reacts.

In my last book, I taught you about this response and its effect on our
metabolism, health, and aging. I have been measuring this response for
over twenty years and I discovered that it is the management of this
response that is the real key in creating weight loss, increased energy,
and overall health. Metabolism is energy and there really isn't such a
thing as a 'bad metabolism.' I have discovered that the metabolism is

either working or it isn't. A working metabolism will burn fat for energy.

When there is an imbalance in the body it stores fuel (fat) and we gain weight. Not only do we gain weight but also our body breaks down and begins to age faster which leads to all the lifestyle diseases such as heart disease and diabetes. The key to wellness, age management and permanent weight loss lies in the body's ability to recuperate from each day. The key becomes the management of the stress response, a survival response that we cannot shut off.

In clinics that I've been involved with, we have taken 70-year-old diabetics and reversed the disease. How? Simple. We create a program of recuperation and the body begins to repair itself on a daily basis and like magic we take control of their health. Here is what I have found happens when we control the stress response.

- We begin to sleep more soundly and wake up rested. This is because when the stress response is unmanaged the body stays on guard and keeps the adrenaline flowing to take action if needed. Our body is built for survival and has no idea why you were so stressed during the day. It's as if the body sleeps with one eye open, just in case.

- We think with more clarity and make better decisions. The reason this happens is when we manage stress we manage the part of the nervous system that allows us to respond with clarity.

- Our energy levels are high and consistent. We do not have those energy ups and downs. The reason for higher energy is when we manage the stress response our body will use fat for energy and this allows us to manage the brain's fuel (sugar) throughout the day. When our sugar levels drop our energy levels follow.

- We lose cravings for carbohydrates and sugar. When we manage the stress response we manage our energy and sugar levels. When stress goes unmanaged our sugar drops and we experience cravings for sweets or carbohydrates.

Throughout the years people have commented on how disciplined I was. I never seemed to break my program no matter what the situation was. I wish I could tell you that I had this super-magic pill that made me follow my diet and get out of bed and exercise. The truth is I am a compulsive overeater and I am genetically from a family with obesity.

No, my success has nothing to do with me being disciplined; it's all about the system I have created.

My system is geared to manage the stress response—the key in having a healthy fat-burning metabolism.

The stress response is one of nature's greatest gifts to mankind: the built-in ability of your body and brain to devote all of its energy to fight-or-flight from an emergency. The stress response does not waste energy—physical or mental—on anything that does not help you survive the immediate crisis. So when the fight-or-flight response takes over, the physical energy that might a moment ago have been devoted to digesting a meal or recuperating from yesterday's workout is redirected to the task of immediate self-preservation. Mental energy that was focused on solving the challenge with your company's budget is rechanneled into present-moment vigilance and rapid action. In other words, the fight-or-flight stress response is an energy-management instinct. It decides how you are going to spend your limited physical and mental energy. The stress response cannot be shut off; only managed. When it is not managed we will crave sweets, procrastinate, be reactive and live a life in a constant anxious state of being. Even more pressing is the fact that when the stress response is running hot we become compulsive and all self-control goes out the window.

When we manage the stress response we lose weight and experience incredible energy. You won't have food cravings and you will feel motivated to make better decisions without being pressed. In other words, you have more self-control. The reason is you stimulate the part of the nervous system that allows discipline and self-control and this is the other survival response, the pause-plan response.

Pause-Plan Response

I have seen thousands of patients in our clinics over these last few years, allowing me to test the stress response in a large demographic cross-section of patients. We have had incredible success in helping patients lose weight and become healthy by managing their stress response; even patients in their seventies and eighties have become success stories. We have such a great track record of getting patients off their medications that we only use medicine as a tool to stabilize the patient because we know that our wellness program will heal the metabolism and they won't need the medicine any longer. My challenge over these last few years was to really figure it out—why did patients fail? We know that the program we are giving them is geared to their unique physiology and it will work. Yet patients will fail and quit, even after losing 30 to 40 pounds.

I have spent years researching the science of self-discipline. I discovered incredible works being done in this area. Here is a list of credible researchers to follow; Dr. Roy Baumeister, Dr. Daniel Amen, Rick Hanson, Helen Fisher, Amy Cuddy, Kelly McGonigal, Linda Graham, Susan Segerstrom, Dr. Bruce Lipton, Dr. Rick Harris. I am so excited by all that I have discovered in the science of discipline and I am even more amazed by my daily rituals that I have created over the years that have had a direct effect on my personal discipline.

So what was this incredible discovery? That there is actually an opposing response to the stress response and it is called the *pause-plan response*. Suzanne Segerstrom, a psychologist at the University of Kentucky, studies how states of mind like stress and hope influence the body. She has found that, just like stress, self-control has a biological signature. The need for self-control sets into motion a coordinated set of changes in the brain and body that helps you resist temptation and override self-destructive urges by activating the self-control mechanism. Segerstrom calls those changes the pause-and-plan response, which couldn't look more different from the fight-or-flight response. The pause-plan response runs directly opposite of the stress response, and the management of stress has a direct effect on the pause-plan response.

The stress response activates the brain and body to go into survival mode to fight or flee. This can be very challenging when you are stuck in traffic and the driver in front of you cuts you off causing you to slam on your brakes, and then proceeds to flip you the bird. In most cases all reasoning goes out the window as your heart is beating out of your chest and you're getting ready to go kick some butt. With the stress response going off full tilt, what can you do? You could jump out of the car and run down the street or you could attack the other driver but both of these reactions would most likely end badly. Or you could shut the stress response off and turn on the pause-plan response. You can actually turn on the response that will calm you down and shut off the stress response.

The pause-plan response connects you to the self-control regions of the prefrontal cortex of the brain. The prefrontal cortex has been called the CEO of the brain. As you recall, it is the captain (conscious mind). Like the fight-or-flight response, the pause-plan response begins in the brain. Just as the alarm system of your brain is always monitoring what you hear, see, taste, and smell, other areas are keeping track of what is going on inside you. This self-monitoring system is distributed throughout the brain, connecting the self-control regions of the prefrontal cortex with areas of the brain that keep track of your body sensations, thoughts, and emotions.

One important job of this system is to activate self-control that keeps you on your diet and getting up in the morning to go for a walk. When you're tempted to cheat on your diet or procrastinate on an important project that is due, the prefrontal cortex jumps into action to help you make the right choice. To help the prefrontal cortex, the pause-plan response redirects energy from the body to the brain. This is the opposite effect that the stress response has as it directs the energy away from the brain to the lower extremities to take action. For self-control, you do not need legs ready to run or arms ready to punch, but a well-fueled brain to connect to its self-control mechanism to do what needs to be done or not do what should be avoided.

The Responses in Action

Both the stress response and the pause-plan response are components of our survival DNA. They can be stimulated by our emotions and our interpretation of events. In other words, our thoughts can work on either system. The stress response is part of the sympathetic nervous system that stimulates us to react. The pause-plan response is part of the parasympathetic nervous system the puts you and your body in a calm state and allows us to respond. Both responses were crucial for our early survival.

During those times of roaming predators that were looking at humans as a meal, the stress response was there to save us. The moment we eyed that saber-toothed tiger our body immediately went into survival mode. The first step was for the brain to shut down the parasympathetic nervous system meaning the reasoning and responsive part of the brain was turned off. The reason the body does this is because it does not want you to analyze the tiger; it wants you to get the hell out of there! So as the parasympathetic nervous system shuts down, the sympathetic nervous system kicks in with the stress response. When the body's stress response goes off, it's all hands on deck so all the energy is focused on the fight-or-flight reaction. The blood leaves the brain and heads to our extremities along with a flood of adrenaline and it is time for the flight-or-fight response to get us moving toward safety. To ensure there is enough fuel the body shuts down all unnecessary systems such as our immune and digestive systems.

On the other end of the spectrum we needed the pause-plan response to figure out new ways to enhance our lives. We had to pause and plan and think about better ways to live and be able to survive the dangers that surrounded us. We invented fire, tools and ways to work with other humans to create a successful tribe. This took self-control and calm thought of the parasympathetic nervous system. We needed the CEO of the brain, the captain, to direct our actions toward growth.

The challenge we all face today is that our body believes it is still living in the cave, but today's tiger consists of too much traffic, not enough time, information over-load, cell phones, 24-hour news, reality television, and getting the kids to soccer practice on time. When we are sitting in traffic late for our appointment the body cannot tell the difference between that or being chased by the tiger; it *reacts*! Today it seems our stress response is on 24/7, and with that the sympathetic nervous system stays activated causing us anxiety, restless sleep, depression and a host of other metabolic disturbances that cause weight gain, heart disease, diabetes, etc. Even more important, while the stress response sympathetic nervous system is firing, our pause-plan parasympathetic is shut down. In other words, the brain's CEO has left the building. When this happens not only are we stressed to the limits but also our self-control mechanism is turned off causing us to break every resolution we set for ourselves.

The Challenge of Self-Control

You have made your New Year's resolution to get back into shape. You have a set program to exercise six days a week, cut sugar from your diet and not eat past 7 p.m. each night. You have meticulously planned your healthy assault by getting rid of all the holiday junk food and plan to wake up at 6 a.m. and walk your dog to ensure you get in the exercise.

It all starts out well, your enthusiasm gets you through the first two weeks and you actually started to do 45 minutes on the treadmill to go along with the dog walking. At this point you have lost seven pounds and then it happens; the fatigue starts in, and excuses begin to make their appearance and the routine starts to become challenging. (*Note: This is the Snap Back Effect of the 30-day Comfort Zone Testing Period.*)

You begin to get more and more discouraged and frustrated with yourself. You begin to hit the snooze alarm and breaking your diet with the promise that you will start again tomorrow. This is perhaps your tenth attempt at weight loss over the last few years and every time the scene unfolds the same way—with self-sabotage.

Each diet you begin with a great deal of zest and zeal but within the first month what began as a well-planned effort to change falls into meaningless justifications for self-sabotage. I have no discipline, no self-control; I can't even get out of bed when I want in the morning let alone keep up with an exercise program. I have bad genetics and I can't live without carbs plus I'm too busy to eat so early and my husband won't support me. The more this pattern happens the worse the self-esteem becomes. "Why can't I have self-control and be disciplined? Why am I so weak? I hate myself."

The truth is there is a science to properly creating and keeping resolutions. The scientific evidence of self-control shows that discipline takes energy and that energy supply is not endless. If the discipline energy supply runs low then the self-control mechanism shuts off and we are off to the bingeing races.

Dr. Kelly McGonigal's writes in her book *The Willpower Instinct* about the research of Dr. Roy Baumeister, a research scientist at Florida State University, who compares our willpower to a muscle. Just as a muscle needs to be exercised, rested, nourished and challenged, so must our willpower for it to be strong and effective. We have to work at managing the stress response and building our prefrontal cortex to strengthen the pause-plan response.

I have told people that my greatest secret in keeping off 100 pounds for over thirty years is that I cheat. The Junk Night link was discovered when I was getting ready for my first bodybuilding contest and I snapped and went on a binge.

It is essential that you understand that self-control is about building and activating the pause-plan response parasympathetic nervous system but it is also about managing the stress response sympathetic nervous system. Self-control is not just a mindset; it is a physiological process involving the mind and body along with the survival responses. We must understand that self-discipline is a mind-body response to any external challenge. When you use your willpower you are using energy in the brain and when this energy fails you sabotage your efforts. It's like continuing exercise beyond your fitness level and continuing to push your body, either you burnout or pass out from exhaustion. If you are trying to change too many things that require your willpower you will crash and burn. But, on the other hand if you are training to get in better shape you have to push your body past your comfort zone and keep training even when you'd rather quit and go home to slump in front of the television. The self-control mechanism grows when you pass on instant gratification and stay on course of your personal development challenge. *The Ten Minute Life Plan* techniques are self-control exercises to build the self-control muscle.

If we look at self-control in the context of exercise, the ability to keep long term goals or changes in mind is important while pursuing an activity that may or may not in that moment, be an enjoyable experience. In fact it may be quite uncomfortable. You must have a strong purpose— a strong *why*—so when the Snap Back Effect occurs you keep going. Weight loss results are never instantaneous; it requires months of work and consistency to make lifestyle changes. I can tell you from personal experience that you must train the self-control mechanism and reprogram your comfort zone in order to create permanent changes. I could easily gain my weight back because of my genetics, but I control my genetics with my daily habits. The key to successful personal development is doing the work in order to manage the survival responses. If stress goes unmanaged the self-control mechanism is shut down. This is why so many people ride the personal development rollercoaster.

Chapter Four: Procrastination; I Will Start Tomorrow

My advice is to never do tomorrow what you can do today. Procrastination is the thief of time. — Charles Dickens

While working in personal development I notice that people believe there are actually magic days to start a diet, or exercise program, or to quit smoking, or to start a budget, or to work on their relationship. New Year's Day is a magical day of change. Diet programs are booming, gym memberships are growing, and Anthony Robbins cannot keep his programs in stock. If you are like most people January first turns into January 8th, which then eases on into January 15th—and then you may or may not start. This is a pattern I have seen each New Year without fail. Another great day to start changing is our birthday. We swear that this year will be different and we will lose that weight and get back into a closet of clothes that no longer fit. The most used day to create change is Monday! People love to start their programs on Monday. Of course it seems that every Monday they are starting over.

I have wondered my entire career why we procrastinate on such important things as our health or life dream? I can tell you this that my most successful clients are the ones who just suffered a heart attack or just got diagnosed with diabetes. They beg me to give them the answers to change their life. In my *Stress Mastery* courses, I teach Ten Success Principles and Seven Steps that are basically tools to get people to do the work of finding a mission—a purpose—for the change they wish to generate. To change a habit and create the life we want we must take consistent action outside the comfort zone and have a strong *why* to fight the Snap Back Effect. But we procrastinate for several reasons and the most scientific reason is we are not managing our energy levels and the stress response well. To change we must do the work and yes, step outside our comfort zone. For this to happen with the consistency that is needed to create change, *we must control STRESS!*

The challenge I see in most personal development courses is that they have great tools to motivate us to get started, but they lack the understanding of the stress role when it comes to activating the self-control mechanism in the brain. We have to have discipline in order to use the tools they teach. On the other hand we can have a great lifestyle program of diet and exercise but we lack the tools of personal development to prevent the Snap Back Effect and reprogram the comfort zone. As I have stated before, I never really created changes in my body until I started studying personal development and combining my studies into the working metabolism. Now with the study of willpower, self-discipline, and brain health everything is now coming together.

The System of Discipline: Red Zone/Green Zone

Rick Hanson, Ph.D., is a neuropsychologist and New York Times best-selling author. His books include *Hardwiring Happiness*, *Buddha's Brain*, *Just One Thing*, and *Mother Nurture*. He is the Founder of the Wellspring Institute for Neuroscience and Contemplative Wisdom. Dr. Hanson has a spectacular way of referring to the survival responses as **Red Zone** and **Green Zone.**

Dr. Hanson refers to the "responsive mode of the brain as the pause-plan mode of the Green Zone." At the other end of the spectrum the "reactive mode of the brain is referred to as the stress response mode of the Red Zone." Mother Nature has endowed us with both settings in the brain: the *reactive* setting, where we experience our most fundamental needs of safety, satisfaction, and connection. When the brain fires up into its fight or flight stress *response* mode or goes into an intense freeze mode, it activates the Red Zone. While in the Red Zone (which is not meant to be sustainable at all as it is manifested as a brief burst), the body burns resources faster than it takes them in. Bodily systems are really disturbed. There is a fundamental sense of deficit and disturbance, and long-term building projects like strengthening the immune system and digestion are put on hold.

My coaching and wellness programs are built to manage the two survival zones. In *Shift Coaching,* I use Ten Success Principles to reprogram the comfort zone with new habits of thinking and taking action. But, the key to everything Green is managing the Red and the stress response. The stress response is designed for a short period of escaping a dangerous situation and then it's to default to the pause-plan response where we recuperate, create and live in touch with our higher purpose. If we live our lives without managing the stress response we then live our life in the Red Zone. I have found once my clients hit age 45, and especially as they hit their fifties, many actually get stuck in the Red Zone. When the Red Zone is activated the Green Zone is shut down causing deterioration in mental and physical health. In *TRUTH* the entire purpose of the book is to educate you on a lifestyle that manages these two survival responses.

Another interesting fact that research is showing is that managing the two nervous systems is the key to self-discipline, self-control and willpower. The sympathetic nervous system is reactive and directly in connection with the ***Stress Response (Red Zone).*** The parasympathetic nervous system is responsive and directly in connection with the ***Pause-Plan Response (Green Zone).*** The action we take or don't take is directly linked to the management of these zones.

Everyone seems to think I have a magic pill of self-discipline. In my career I travel the world lecturing plus I have a busy social life associated with my work. I never cheat on my program. The key word here is program. As I stated earlier I live a system that is designed to balance the stress response and connect to the pause-plan response. I never cheat on my program but I do cheat on my diet every week and have been cheating for over thirty years. Also my system includes a diet built for my physiology designed for maximum recuperation and stress response management. We cannot shut off the stress response but we can manage it allowing us to switch on the pause-plan response. You will still have stressful situations in your life and the world isn't going to slow down but you can easily activate your *Green Zone* with simple techniques.

When I exercise I want one result and that is increased Heart Rate Variability (HRV). HRV is the measurement of the heart rate when you breathe-in and breathe-out. The higher the variability or the number of beats the better. When you have a high HRV it means that your heart is getting signals from both branches of your autonomic nervous system: the sympathetic nervous system (the stress response), which revs the body into action, and the parasympathetic nervous system (the pause-plan response), which promotes relaxation and healing in the body. I accomplish this because my exercise program is built into the system from testing. I know the exact intensity and amount of exercise I need for maximum recuperation. I have been measuring heart rate for twenty-five years, educating the importance of making exercise more precise. I never train without monitoring my heart rate but even more important is to know the correct heart rate zones for your body. If we exercise too hard for our body's ability to recuperate we then decrease HRV. In other words, we stress our body in such a way that it turns on the Red Zone, which leads to a shutdown of the self-control mechanism. Simply put, the no pain, no gain workout you did this morning will lead to thinking it's ok to have that pint of Ben and Jerry's sitting in the freezer tonight.

In my system I also have consistent personal development tools that include everything from regular meditation to a clear purpose to daily journaling. I use sleep cycles and sleep with meditation mp3 in my ears all night. I also take supplements that my body needs to work at an optimal level and most important I actively test my blood, Vo2 Max and work hand-in-hand with my doctor. This is the system that creates my lifestyle that keeps me disciplined. It's not the discipline that keeps the system.

The Energy of Discipline

The human brain and the stress response are wired for us to take appropriate action in any given situation where we are in danger. It is important to remember that our body is really only designed for one thing and that is survival. Our brain is also set up to survive and does this by conserving energy. That is why we have a comfort zone and every event we experience the brain works to put it into a category (habits) so it does not have to think or analyze. The less the brain has to work the more energy it has reserved for when it needs to perform a fight-or-flight action or to figure out an answer to a complicated problem. Our brain uses a large amount of energy—20% of our energy—on a regular basis though it only accounts for 2% of our body weight.

So, let's take a closer look at the stress response in action and how it uses our energy reserves. You're going for a nice nature walk through the woods and you come face to face with a bear. Your body is going to react in a hurry. The stress response fires and all your energy and impulses are for you to flee as fast as possible. The brain immediately shuts down the parasympathetic nervous system and the pause-plan response, putting the body on automatic pilot. The muscles want to run faster than ever before, your heart is beating through your chest, adrenaline is pouring into the bloodstream as cortisol spikes to pull-up quick sugar for some ready to go fuel. Meanwhile the body shuts down anything not needed to fight-or-flight from the situation. All rational thought goes out the window as reactive thought of getting the hell out of here takes over. The stomach stops all digestion, as the blood is needed to hit our lower limbs so we can move quickly, as the breath increases to get oxygen to these muscles. We are ready to fight to the death or take off like a bat out of hell. But WAIT, it isn't a bear! It's a bunch of twigs wrapped in a bush that looks just like a bear. Relief, yes but the sympathetic nervous system has your body high as a kite on adrenaline and no place to go.

Today this scenario plays out in all kinds of ways all throughout the day. The stress response was the appropriate response to get away from the bear, but it's not appropriate when you have to give a talk in front of people, or when you ask someone out on a date, or when you are stuck in traffic and late for an appointment. You can clearly see my point in today's modern world. We live in a stressed out society and our poor body is in complete reaction mode. We are built to survive in a cave, not in traffic or with 24-hour news access and technology.

So, what does this stressed out state have to do with self-control and procrastination? Everything! The main fuel for the stress response is glucose, which happens to be the main fuel for the self-control response of pause-plan. When your glucose levels get low and you are low on energy it is highly likely that you will avoid or give up on any given task much more easily. This blood sugar drop is one of the main reasons that we will lose our self-control.

Over the years I have found that when I have a client and we manage their stress response they cease to have cravings for sweets and they feel energetic toward exercising. The moment the client misses a snack everything unravels so at night their diet usually ends in a binge. In other words, complete loss of self-control and willpower.

The bottom-line to self-control and creating any type of self-discipline we must manage the stress response so we manage our energy levels. But, it has also been shown that an act that requires any type of self-discipline and requires the use of the parasympathetic pause-plan response also uses glucose. If you are resisting that bowl of candy, trying to be good on your diet, you will use your self-control energy supply and this could make you procrastinate on other important work that may be due.

Do you know of people who have stopped smoking and then start eating? Started a diet and began spending money? It seems that one act of self-control then leads to an act of self-indulgence, or to the act of procrastination. The one key factor in all of this is blood sugar management.

Brain Energy Conversation

The brain loves to make connections and 'hardwire' everything. This is related to a variety of factors. First, the brain likes to stay in a state of homeostasis thus the need for the comfort zone. The brain does not want to waste energy with creating any type of change. Second, it takes energy (glucose) for the brain to process information in its workings, and our body is great at storing fat while not so great at storing glucose. Third, the brain likes to conserve this energy. The way it conserves energy is by putting everything into a category. This is why new ideas are usually met with resistance. Brain categories become habits allowing us to be able to operate on autopilot with respect to that activity. Think of any basic activity you learned—walking, brushing your teeth, tying your shoelaces, driving a car—all of them required lots of focus, attention, and energy on the front-end until you learned the skill. Now you can do those things without much thought or effort at all.

Anytime the brain faces new input, it wants to connect it with the existing maps or wiring. Anything that does not fit requires energy for the brain to process and this includes executing any type of disciplined action.

The moment we start any type of personal development we are tapping into our brain's energy. The simple reason is we are stepping outside our comfort zone and taking new actions. Whether it's a new diet, budget or learning a new language the brain needs to use its energy supply. The secret is managing the Red Zone and flipping the Green Zone into action. Procrastination is more than us being lazy; it's also about our built in survival response.

To change we must do the work and take action. To do this we must manage stress and its response on our energy reserves. We must understand the comfort zone and our innate ability to seek survival overrides all good intentions. *The Ten Minute Life Plan* gives you a quick guide and techniques to master procrastination.

Chapter Five: Introducing
The Seven Steps to Stress Mastery

The Seven Steps to Stress Mastery

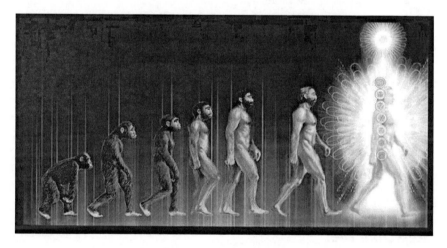

Stress is never going away and the stress response is never shutting off, so management is the only option. **The challenge we have is that we are built for survival, and unfortunately, our survival DNA is still back in the cave.** Our body does not know we are living in modern times, and we are not built for handling traffic, 24-hour news or technology. The challenge is that a large part of today's population is stuck 24-7 in the Red Zone, creating conditions of chronic stress.

The seven-step process is based on the science of stress and the bodies purpose of survival. But, true Stress Mastery leads us to the higher realms where science transitions to spiritual higher consciousness work. People can debate all they want but those who accomplish all seven steps to Stress Mastery achieve a level of success and peace that few ever comprehend. The reason I am writing *The Seven Steps to Stress Mastery* is because I believe this is our birthright for each and every one of us. These steps are the perfect guide; each step creates its own level of change.

What does Stress Mastery look like?

- Stability in mood, calmness and centeredness
- Happier, more consistent sense of ease
- Better self-esteem
- Feeling more in control and able to perform work
- Usual anxiety triggers are no longer an effect
- Higher / more stable energy
- Ease of digestion
- Free of aches & pains
- Better circulation
- Higher adaptability and ability to solve problems
- More ease integrating learning experiences
- Improved libido
- Higher focus
- Clearer thinking and decision-making
- Better ability to take on work and tasks
- Appetite regulation
- Overall peaceful state

Step One: Diet

The stress response never shuts off and the first step in mastering stress starts with our diet. The body is built for survival and fat is our survival fuel. The diet rules are quite simple, and in my new book, you will be taught how to conduct your own experiment on your body using the stages of eating. Our body talks to us through its signals of craving. The main thing to understand with our diet is that the stress response responds to the diet in a balanced or unbalanced manner. The two things that disrupt the stress response are not eating in a timely manner and sugar.

The Stress Response

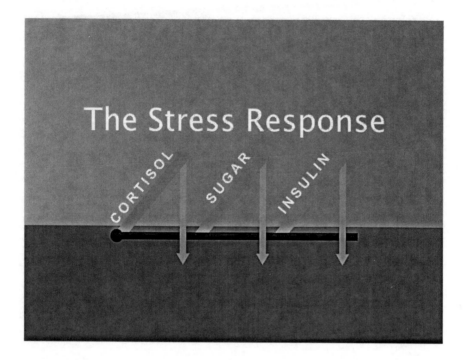

The response is triggered by any situation that we perceive as dangerous. It is also triggered when we experience any type of change, and it doesn't matter if the change is good for us or not. Finally, the stress response is triggered if someone or something activates one of your subconscious programs. These include your values and all your beliefs.

So, if you believe that the boss is going to be upset because you are late, the stress response fires, and it fires as if you are in life or death danger. The stress hormones release, being led by the cortisol hormone. This signals the body that it needs fuel to fight or flight. The body then brings up its sugar levels, which is the fuel the body uses in stress situations. The body then releases the insulin hormone.

Sugar and the Stress Response

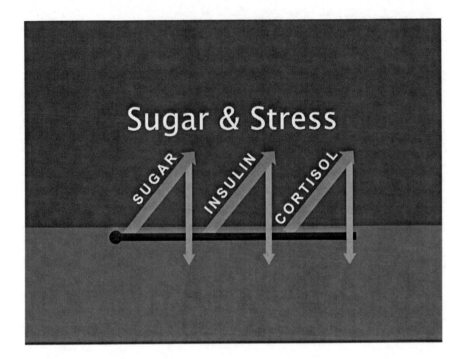

The diet is key in managing stress and a bad diet is the kiss of death when it comes to stress management. Not eating breakfast, going too long between meals, not enough protein, all contribute to increased stress and an imbalanced stress response. But, nothing contributes more to stress than sugar. Sugar comes from all types of carbohydrates: grains, fruits, alcohol—they all turn to sugar. **If your body does not process sugar, the moment you consume any type of carbohydrate, you will experience an imbalanced stress response.**

The big issue with sugar and stress is that it causes a roller coaster effect. The sugar causes the stress response to jump high and then to slam down. **When it's high we feel good for the moment, when it's low we are tired and CRAVE sweets and carbs.** Thus, we crave more sugar and the whole process starts over. When the stress response is jumping up and down, the nervous system stays stuck in the Red Zone. You CANNOT burn fat in the Red Zone.

Step Two: Exercise

Exercise is rather confusing when it comes to managing stress as exercise is a form of stress. The right exercise is exercise that your body can recuperate from. **If you exercise too hard then the body will get stuck in the Red Zone and have low cortisol hormone levels.** The balance of the cortisol hormone is essential for recuperation and well-being. Some of us are born to lift weights and others are to run. It's like at the race track where you have the pace car going around the track at a nice slow pace, and then the car veers off and the race cars take off. Exercise is essential but you need to know if you are a pacer or a racer. It comes down to the management of the cortisol hormone that drives the stress response.

Cortisol Hormone

In medicine, the Cortisol hormone is very misunderstood. The reference ranges are from really low to high, and basically tell you nothing. Cortisol cascades throughout the day so it is supposed to start high in the morning and then start dropping mid-morning, still lower by mid-afternoon to its lowest point in the evening.

When you test Cortisol, you are not looking for illness, you are looking at stress. Cortisol's job is to prepare the body to start the day. It is high in the morning for this reason, and one of its main functions is to increase serotonin in the brain. Serotonin makes us feel happy and ready to face the day. **Low A.M. Cortisol results in low serotonin, which results in depression.**

Some people who run hot (high stress) have the Cortisol cycle reversed where it's high at night and low in the morning, and will have issues with sleep. Cortisol is also our body's natural anti-inflammatory; too low we get aches and pains, too high we get muscle breakdown.

Step Three: Naming the Ego

Our daily actions come from the programming installed in our sub-conscious mind. This programming is designed never to change and is protected by the comfort zone cage. The subconscious programs hold all our values, beliefs, and habits and these are what make up our self-concept or ego.

Every action we take or don't take, every habit both good or bad, come from the operating system of the subconscious mind. The challenge we have is that many of our programs come during the first seven years of life. This process is what I call Tribalization, and it is another of our survival mechanisms. Tribalization is designed to get us to fit into our culture, society, religion, and most importantly, into the tribes' beliefs as fast as possible. Once these programs are installed, they are designed to never be uninstalled and they make up who you believe you are.

These programs cause us to stress out and react. In step three, you begin developing self-awareness, and this is the first step in re-setting your mind's operating system. **In this step, you begin separating YOU from the concept of who you think you are, and this process begins to calm the nervous system towards the Green Zone.**

Step Four: Letting Go

When we get to step four, we are now managing the stress response and developing awareness of that voice in our head. It is in this step that we can now actively start resetting our operating system of the subconscious mind. It is the technique that we learn in this step that allows us to change long-time habits and limiting beliefs. **The art of letting go of old programs begins to raise our conscious energy levels.** When these levels raise, two distinct things begin to happen. First, we've broken old habits and patterns; second, we now are attracting new incredible things, people and situations into our lives.

Step Five: Green Focus Power Hour

The Green Focus Power Hour (GFPH) is a powerful tool that is designed for the advance reset of the subconscious Cage. It is a series of exercises that are performed in the morning to replace old programs and set your day to start in the Green Zone. **It is the GFPH that begins transitioning you toward the more spiritual side of the Stress Mastery process.** The GFPH can have incredible impacts on one's life in as little as 30-days. Step five will give you a lifetime tool to set each day in the Green Zone, which is the key in Stress Mastery.

Step Six: Meditation

We've all seen the studies on how meditation has a positive effect on all aspects of wellness and longevity. But the true purpose of meditation is to develop the art of concentration. It is mastering this art that brings you truly to Stress Mastery. **Meditation has two very distinct purposes in Stress Mastery: first, to connect us to the superconscious mind which brings everything in our lives, and second, to separate us from our ego.** Meditation is the tool that strengthens the self-awareness muscle.

Meditation, done properly, will flip the nervous system from Red Zone to Green Zone. Once developed, meditation is a tool that can be used at anytime, anywhere. We can literally flip from Red to Green in a matter of seconds. As one nears Stress Mastery, meditation becomes easier and much more predominate in our lives as we are now going from science to spirit in our life's journey.

Step Seven: Finding the NOW

Step seven is where we live the three-step spiritual practice. Step one is to be present and live in the moment. **It is in the NOW where we master stress because we no longer are concerned about the past or future.** Step two is self-awareness, and this is the moment that you noticed you were pulled from the present moment. It's this awareness that allows you to release the program that pulled you out of the moment. This leads to step three, where we surrender to the energy of that program back to the present, NOW.

The three-step practice is taking place all throughout the day, and it's this practice that takes us to the surrendered conscious energy. It's this energy where you experience Stress Mastery. It is simply a state of peace. You no longer see good and bad, you just experience the event. It is an incredible state that is hard to put into words.

Simply put, Stress Mastery is peace.

Chapter Six: The Ten Minute Life Plan

A Dozen Techniques to End Procrastination... In Ten Minutes or Less!

Technique One: Diet

The *TRUTH* is if you don't manage your diet you cannot manage the stress response and the Red Zone. The simple approach to diet is this technique to manage the Red Zone. Basically if you manage your sugar levels you manage the stress response. Here are three easy diet steps to get you started today.

- Cut the sugar is my first and foremost advice. Just cutting the sugar out will dramatically improve your energy and focus.

- Eat breakfast. Make sure you have a protein which is the key food in managing the Red Zone. This meal should consist of a healthy grain, low glycemic fruit, and a protein (bowl of oatmeal with blueberries and a scoop of whey protein).

- Eat small meals every three hours. If you go too long between meals or if you skip meals the Red Zone fires up. When this happens the Green Zone shuts down and we usually binge and overeat unhealthy foods.

- Whey protein drink between meals is the easiest and best way to manage our stress response. I have seen in the diabetics I work with that if they take a whey protein drink between meals their sugar levels will drop even if they didn't make any other dietary changes. Whey protein has been a huge component in my life and all my programs.

Technique Two: Ten-Minute Timer Exercise

One of my favorite techniques to overcome procrastination is the ten-minute timer exercise. I use this technique personally and with all my coaching clients. *When we start any type of personal development the comfort zone is strongest in the first 30 days.* It is essential that we take action and do the work that must be done in order to create the desired change. The comfort zone uses procrastination as a way to knock you out of a routine or keep you from an action that is not programmed in the subconscious (your habits). The secret is consistency to break an old program and to establish a new program. Set the timer for ten minutes and use it in two ways.

- **The "I WONT" Response.** With my clients that are trying to break bad habits such as eating sweets after dinner, compulsive shopping, smoking, gossiping, etc. I use the "I won't" response. Here is how it works: Say you are rolling along and doing fantastic on your new diet plan. You've had your dinner and the kids are fed but there is a brownie on the counter. You eye that brownie and all your instincts are yelling for you to attack! The voice in your head says, *"It's ok, you exercised this morning and have been perfect on your eating plan."* You scream NO! Well, maybe one bite? My mother always told me it's ok to have a little. But, I can have it on Junk Night, Right? Every dieter has faced that moment of truth. Most of us will try to just take a bite, but then what the heck, we may as well eat the whole thing. Many times once we have given in then we say to ourselves, "I will start back on my diet again in the morning" and then proceed to eat five brownies.

  - ✓ *The Ten-Minute I WONT response works like this:* You want the brownie but in order for you to have it you have a set rule. *You set your timer for ten minutes and pull out your journal.* Write anything that is on your mind, most likely you will write about the brownie, I know, duh. After the ten minute timer goes off if you still want the brownie then have at it. When it comes to changing eating habits this technique has worked wonders on my clients. The simple act of journaling turns on the Green Zone where it's easy to say NO.

- **The "I WILL" Response.** I personally use this technique pretty much on a daily basis. When I have several projects at the same time the first thing that seems to be put on the wayside is my writing. The hardest thing about writing a book is sitting down and writing it. Once I start writing I fall in love with the process. It's the starting part that will get me every time. I have spoken to several authors and they say the same thing. The reason for this is the *comfort zone resistance*. The same thing happens with any new undertaking such as exercise, hobbies, any personal development, or budget keeping. The voice in the head usually says *I will do it later* or *I will start tomorrow, I promise*. Most of us experienced this when we were given a school project and a two-month notice of when it will be due. Yes, we start it the day before and work all night killing our self to get it done. Any type of work that you have told yourself you are going to do and you find yourself putting it off is perfect for the I Will Response.

  ✓ *The Ten Minute I WILL Response works like this:* Set your timer for ten minutes and then sit down and do the work. The key is you only have to do it for the ten-minute period; once the timer goes off you are done. Or maybe you decide to continue to work a little longer. The key to change is consistent action. It does not matter that it was only ten minutes. The subconscious cannot tell time. This is a great tool for starting an exercise program, personal development exercises such as journaling, meditation, and working on three or more projects at a time. It is the most amazing act of how ten minutes turns into a productive 1 or 2 hours of work. Or the work may end after the timer rings and you have stayed on a consistent track of progress.

Technique Three: Two-Minute Posture/Presence Reset

Posture, the way you carry yourself, is one of your most important assets in creating a first impression. Do you project youth, vigor, power, confidence and style when you enter a room? Does your body language say, "Look at me"? Your carriage is cosmetically as important as good hair and clothes are. Presence is a person's bearing, especially when it comes to commanding a respectful attention. It is the quality of self-assurance and effectiveness that permits someone to achieve great results no matter what the undertaking. What happens to the energy in a room when you enter? Do you command attention? Do people gravitate to you?

Posture/Presence is a success tool that will not only portray to the outside world that you are a winner but also to your inner self that you are a star.

When that inner self-image gets the positive message then everything changes. Posture and presence are aspects over which you have control. This is about being aware of how you are feeling and how you are carrying yourself in that moment. Whatever the situation act as if you have already succeeded. Simply put, *fake it until you make it!* The other great effect from acting in this manner is that you change over the Red Zone to the Green Zone and your change in posture actually changes your physiology.

Harvard social psychologist Amy Cuddy has documented how positive and negative body language shapes your self-perception and your hormone levels. In Cuddy's experiment done in collaboration with Dana Carney at Berkeley, one group spent two minutes doing low power poses—head down, shoulders sunk, eyes averted, and looking small. The other group did high-power poses—hands on hips, chest lifted, staring boldly out at the horizon a la Wonder Woman. Then they took a saliva sample. The high-power posers showed a nearly 20 percent increase in testosterone (the dominance hormone) and a 25 percent decrease in cortisol (the stress hormone). The low-power posers saw a 10 percent decline in testosterone and a 17 percent increase in cortisol. Cuddy says, "These two-minute changes (in the body stance) lead to hormonal changes that can configure your brain to be either assertive, confident and comfortable, or really stress reactive and feeling shut down."

Use these simple methods throughout the day anytime you feel tired or uninspired. In two minutes you will have renewed energy and confidence to handle any situation. Here are some sample poses:

1. **Superman or Wonder Woman Pose.** Stand tall, head high with your hands on your hips and assume the posture of your super-

hero. Hold that pose and feel the power for two minutes. Affirm, *"I am strong and powerful!"*

2. **Victory Pose.** Hold your arms above your head as if you just broke the tape at the finish line of a big race. Hold the pose for two minutes. Affirm, *"I am a winner!"*

3. **Smile Pose.** Look in the mirror and put a huge smile on your face. Hold the smile for two minutes. Affirm, *"I am happy and I feel great!"* Note you can do this without a mirror anytime you feel down. I love doing the Smile Pose in traffic it calms me down and it can be entertaining to the car next to me.

Technique Four: Journaling

One of the success principles in my coaching program and in the new book *TRUTH* is journaling. Many times when we get overwhelmed or experience a negative situation we will get stuck in the Red Zone. In other words, we get stuck in a negative attitude program and we keep playing the negative theme over and over. When this happens we release the stress hormones and shut down the responsive Green Zone, only making the challenge seem even bigger as we are in a reactive mode. One of the fastest ways to flip the switch on the Red Zone is to write.

Most of us have had the experience of really being upset at someone and writing them a letter. While you are writing you pour your anger into the words on the paper. Once finished with the letter you feel a sense of relief. Most times as you finish you will sit back and take a deep breath and feel much lighter. By writing out the feelings that were pent up you shut down the reactive mode and switched to the calm responsive mode. In other words, you have switched the Red Zone off and flipped on the Green Zone.

When we get stuck in the Red Zone we procrastinate, complain, experience energy drain, feel anxiety, worry and fear. Journaling is one of the most powerful tools we can use. Here are a couple easy methods that work wonders.

1. Use the timed "I Will" response and Journal for ten minutes to end each day. This can be done before you leave work or before you go to bed. Basically write about anything that is on your mind. Especially pay attention if you are procrastinating on any

type of work that you know needs to be done. Focus in on why you are putting the work off!

2. Use a gratitude journal. Many of us get stuck in the Red Zone because we focus on what we don't have and what is not working. Start each day by writing down ten things that you are grateful for. Examine the things we take for granted like our health, the air we breathe, our family, etc. I start each day with my gratitude journal because it starts my day in the Green Zone.

Technique Five: Breathing

Ok, I know you are breathing but are you breathing or hyperventilating? Maybe that seems like an extreme but it is actually true. When we are in the Red Zone our breath shortens and becomes more rapid in order to prepare us for action. The physiology of the stress response is all about getting the body in a reactive mode to fight or flight. *When we incorporate mindfulness breathing we can immediately shut down the Red Zone and turn on the Green Zone.* This technique can be used anytime and anyplace. Here are a couple simple methods to implement this technique.

1. **Breath Count.** The key in the breathing technique is the exhalation because the exhalation breaths are directly connected to the Green Zone. Take a deep breath in and let it out. On the next breath inhale to a count of ten. As you breathe in count slowly 1 through 10. Then hold the breath for a count of ten. Then exhale slowly to a count of ten. Repeat this pattern for two minutes or as long as it takes until you feel the calm of the Green Zone. This is a great technique before working on a project or even before entering a meeting.

2. **Breathing Through a Straw.** The Green Zone is activated during the exhalation of the breath; the less breaths we take per minute the calmer our state. Take a deep breath in and imagine that you are exhaling slowly thru a straw. The goal is to get our breaths down to 6 to 8 per minute. So, breathe in deep and release slowly for at least two minutes.

Technique Six: Positive Focus Alarms

Many times life can move at a very fast pace and we can get stuck in certain patterns. When we get stuck in a negative pattern we turn on the Red Zone and experience anxiety and stress. As long as we are stuck we will procrastinate or self-sabotage our efforts to grow. One technique that I have utilized over the past several years is setting notices that pop up and remind me to be positive. I have these alarms set up at all different times of the day on my phone. When they appear it causes me to change my focus. It's a friendly reminder that we can choose a positive focus for any situation. I have twelve different messages that go off during the day.

Here are a few examples but make sure the alarm resonates with you personally.

1. Now
2. I Believe
3. Good Things Begin To Happen Now!
4. All Is Well
5. I Am Success
6. I Am A Winner
7. I Am Perfectly Guided
8. I Am A Star
9. I Can Choose Peace
10. I Am Calm

Technique Seven: Ten Minute Green Zone Walk

When it comes to exercise it seems everyone has a different theory of what is right. The truth is I have been doing advance exercise testing for twenty years and I have found that when it comes to stress management a little bit of exercise can change your life dramatically, especially when it comes to procrastinating.

A 2009 study by researchers at the University of Exeter, UK, found that walking for fifteen minutes decreased cravings among smokers, and a 2010 study at the University of Virginia found that two weeks of regular exercise induced brain changes that suppressed cravings and reduced drug-seeking behavior in cocaine-addicted rats. The reason for these results is the exercise switched off the Red Zone and turned on the Green Zone. Once we are in the Green Zone we are managing the stress response, which allows us to make responded choices versus reactive choices. Also by turning on the Green Zone we activate the wellness part of our nervous system lowering our heart rate, slowing our breathing and increasing brain function.

In our medical clinics we measure how a patient's body handles stress at rest and how their body handles stress during exertion (exercise). We can witness a body that is totally stressed out at rest and within thirty seconds of low-level exercise the body relaxes. When we are highly stressed our body, even at rest, is like a teakettle boiling (stuck in the Red Zone) and the moment we start to exercise the steam lets out and the body relaxes (enters the Green Zone). I have watched people change their lives with this simple Green Zone technique. Here are a couple simple ideas to implement this technique.

1. Give yourself 10 minutes or longer to take a walk. Outdoors is best. If weather or obstacles make that impossible use a treadmill or you can actually march in place. Walk at a moderate pace, enough to get your heart rate up slightly. The thing is the Green walk has one purpose and that is to switch the Red Zone over to Green.

2. The Green Zone walk is designed to manage the response and switch us from the Red Zone to the Green Zone. Here are some strategic times to use this technique:

   ✓ **Before Work**. By taking a simple 10-minute walk you get your nervous system ready to roll into the Green Zone and you are ready to start the day with gusto.

   ✓ **Lunch Break**. My coaching clients find that taking a 10-minute walk at midday changes their entire focus. The stress response is more prominent in the afternoon as the day wears on. The Green Zone walk actually refocuses the nervous system to the productive Green Zone. My clients not only report feeling physically much more relaxed but also their productivity increases dramatically.

   ✓ **After Work**. The after work Green walk will not only help you with managing stress but it also can help with your relationships. By taking a simple ten-minute walk around the block before entering the house resets your

> stress response and allows you to respond to your family. By the end of the day most of us have had a tremendous amount of stress and we are stuck in the Red Zone causing us to be in a reactive state of mind. A simple reset allows you to be in a more responsive state of mind to greet your loved ones.

In closing on this technique, I can tell you from years of working with clients that it's by far one of the most effective tools I teach when it comes to managing the stress response. Just think about it. If you follow the technique you will be exercising 30 minutes each day. WOW! SIMPLE!

Technique Eight: Five- to Ten-Minute Meditation

The benefits of meditation are many and varied from reducing stress to increasing one's cognition and creativity. Additionally, meditation heightens our concentration, allowing us to be more productive. This happens because when we meditate we stimulate the Green Zone (parasympathetic nervous system), which strengthens the frontal cortex of the brain. This part of the brain is key to memory, calmness in attitude, recuperation and overall health.

Meditation trains the brain to enter the Green Zone's pause-plan response, which is the opposite of the stress response. Meditation is the exercise for the brain. When we go to the gym and train a muscle the purpose is to increase the muscle size, strength and tone. Meditation does this for the brain. The stronger the prefrontal cortex is the easier it is to flip the nervous system switch from the Red Zone to the Green Zone.

When it comes to meditation most people think that they have to flee to a monastery or spend hours a day sitting in a lotus position to receive these benefits. **Wrong!** It only takes 5 to 10 minutes of mindfulness exercise to create changes in the brain and your overall habit patterns. I personally have meditated for over twenty-five years and I have studied many different theories and techniques. For starting out I recommend the Breathing Meditation but feel free to explore different types of meditations. I find it rather ironic that in the medical field the doctor will tell every patient that they need to exercise and eat better so they can be healthy, but meditation is *just as important and may even be more important as we age*. The reason is simple. As we get older the body doesn't handle stress as well and we can literally get stuck in the Red

Zone or a chronic stressed out state. When this happens our Green Zone is not only shut off but also the prefrontal cortex of the brain actually diminishes.

Eventually if we are stuck in the Red Zone long enough our health, memory and overall quality of life will diminish. The simple technique below will change your life.

Breathing Meditation

This meditation can help you quickly release any unwholesome emotion or stressful situation and bring yourself back into balance whether you are traveling, at work or at home. *The key is to be mindfully aware of your breathing.* To do this you breathe in through your nose for a count of ten, hold for a moment, and then out through your mouth as if you are breathing through a straw, you can choose to count to ten during this exhalation; the important thing is to exhale slowly as this turns on the Green Zone.

Set your timer for the amount of time that you want to do this exercise and then forget about the time. Keep following the routine until you feel comfortable just watching your breath. When you first start this exercise your mind will race with a million thoughts and that is ok. *Your job during meditation is not to shut off the thoughts; it's to be mindful of the thoughts passing through.* In other words, just watch the thought without judgment and focus on the breath. If you find yourself caught up in a thought then simply repeat the ten count upon inhalation and visualize the straw as you breathe out.

It is important that you do not complicate the exercise. Mindfulness training is simply becoming the observer of your mind. Meditation is training for your brain.

Technique Nine: Opposite Hand Diet

Becoming healthy is all about living our lives in the Green Zone. When we manage the stress response Red Zone we can literally change our health immediately. In the Green Zone our body relaxes and wellness takes over as our heart rate lowers, breathing calms, digestion increases, immune system strengthens and our brainpower improves. As we have discussed there are three keys to being in the Green Zone: diet, exercise and mindfulness training. When it comes to diet it is important to eat the right foods, at the right times, in the right combinations, but it's also important to eat mindfully. Mindful eating is the type of eating that many of our parents tried to teach us—slow down and chew your food. I have the tendency to gobble my food down while I am working on something or being distracted by television.

What I call "unmindful eating" is what most of us do on a regular basis as it seems in today's hurry-up world. There just isn't time to stop and eat. What are the consequences of hurried eating? First if you are having a meal and at the same time working or watching the news you are most likely eating in the Red Zone. When we eat in the Red Zone our digestion system is shut down leaving little chance that our body can use the nutrients we just consumed. Also, when we are in the Red Zone the Green Zone shuts down so there is no pause-plan response and we overeat. Finally, if we eat in the Red Zone our metabolisms is in a flight or fight state so we will crave sweets and are more likely to binge on bad foods to end our day. Solution? Simple. Slow down your eating. I know it sounds easy but this simple technique can actually train you to eat more mindfully.

Before we jump into the technique make sure you develop a couple of other eating habits that will reinforce the Green Zone. Do not eat and watch television. Do not eat and work. Don't eat if you are angry or stressed out. Simply pick one of the techniques to change your state before you eat the meal. Finally, try the following technique for a few weeks and see what happens.

Opposite Hand Eating

Simply eat your meals using your opposite hand. I know this technique may sound too simple to work but I promise you in the beginning it is actually not that easy. What it forces you to do is be mindful of what you are eating because if you are not in the moment, you will spill your food. When the pause and plan response is activated with the Green Zone turned on it will cause you to fill up faster and have optimal digestion.

Technique Ten: Notes To The Universe

If I had to pick one specific tool that changed my life more than any other it would be journaling. I have been regularly keeping a journal for the last 34 years. I have written and completed hundreds of journals over the years and have developed some well-tested techniques of journaling. I have found that keeping a day-to-day journal of your experiences, both good and bad, will accelerate your progress toward accomplishing your goals. The reason being is that you can actually see your life experiences unfold as you write. Every week I review my journal to see if there were any patterns, good or bad.

Probably one of the most common reports from people who write journals is that the act of putting thought and feelings on paper helps give useful emotional and mental clarity. However, there is scientific evidence that the relief that comes from writing things down is more than just psychological. Dr. James Pennebaker, a researcher in Texas, has conducted studies that show when people write about emotionally difficult events or feelings for just twenty minutes at a time over three or four days, their immune system's functioning increases. Dr. Pennebaker's studies indicate that the release offered by writing has a direct impact on the body's capacity to withstand stress and fight off infection and disease. The reason this takes place is that we have a tendency to get stuck in the Red Zone dwelling on our problems.

The act of writing clears the subconscious and allows us to switch our nervous system over to the Green Zone where calm and wellness preside. I use several journaling techniques and have found the notes to universe journal is an easy way to manage the survival responses and move us out of neutral, to keep us moving toward what we want.

Notes to the Universe Journal

This is a journal I carry with me at all times. I use a small note pad that fits easily into my pocket. When I want some outcome I will pull this journal out and write to the universe what it is I want. The simple act of writing down an outcome right before you start an activity flips us to the Green Zone so we are responsive and mentally clears anxiety, worry, and any negative thoughts.

I use this technique when I sit down to write, before meetings, events, speaking engagements, anytime I want to get focused quickly. The idea behind this simple journal is to get the universe on my side. I simply take the notebook and write to the universe what I want to happen. Once I write the note I tear the entry off and throw it out. This is my straight communication to God or Universe for guidance. It puts me in the Green Zone state so I can respond to challenges instead of reacting to them.

I have had so many incredible things happen from this tool alone. The simple act of writing it down switches me over from being stressed, to being in the now.

Technique Eleven: Tense and Release

When we are under a lot of stress we can find ourselves stuck in the Red Zone causing us to be in a worried, anxious state. When this happens the body is under constant pressure to react causing it to release a flood of stress hormones that have a profound effect on our whole body. Unmanaged stress causes our muscles to become tight as these hormones change our body's environment. The *tense and release technique* is a quick stress relief tool especially before we go to sleep. Here is a simple guide:

1. Lay down on a bed or a comfortable flat surface. Let the body sink in and take a deep breath in, counting slowly as you inhale to ten. Hold the breath in and count to ten. Slowly release the breath again using the ten count. Repeat this process 3 to 5 times.

2. Once you are semi-relaxed start with the left foot by squeezing it together and holding it for a few seconds then release it. Then flex the calf muscle the same way, holding the tension for a few seconds and then releasing. Work your way to the leg muscle, squeeze and release. Then repeat the same process on the right.

   After you have done both legs follow the same procedure throughout the rest of the body. Squeeze and release the buttocks, abdominal muscles, chest, back, each arm and then finish with the facial muscles and neck area. This whole exercise should take no longer than ten minutes.

3. Once you have completed the Tense and Release technique take a few deep breaths and just relax for a few moments.

Technique Twelve: Subconscious Reset

The subconscious mind is responsible for about 90 percent of the actions we take during any given day. The subconscious programs are the key to success, health and prosperity. When we are actively pursuing any type of personal development we really only have to master two things.

One, we need to work at creating subconscious programs that empower us in our life mission and lead us toward our goals. The second thing is we have to be aware of what we allow into our subconscious mind. We have to be the guard at the gate and the captain of ship. Many of our programs that cause us to procrastinate are fear-based programs that may have been programmed when we were children. But, it is these unconscious programs that will drive you back to the comfort zone the moment you attempt to step out and create change. I use a three-step approach that will help you to reset the subconscious programs. Awareness is the key. The moment that you catch yourself procrastinating, complaining or just feeling uncomfortable simply follow the process listed below.

1. *Feel It.* When you feel uncomfortable or find yourself putting off doing what you know you should be doing, take a moment and feel it. Simply pause, take a breath and ask yourself, "What am I feeling in this moment?"

2. *Release It.* After taking a moment and seeing just what you are feeling try to pinpoint where you feel it and give it a label. For example, I am feeling anxiety and I feel it in my stomach area. Do not complicate this. Once you have identified the feeling take a deep breath and release it to the universe.

3. *Relink the feeling to a positive anchor.* After the release simply replace the feeling with a positive affirmation. I find that the '*I Am...*' affirmations work best with this exercise. Let's say that you had a feeling of anxiety about talking to your boss. After the release simply affirm, "I am strong and confident!" and then go to it.

What this powerful technique does is reprograms the subconscious on the spot. We procrastinate when we step outside the comfort because of our programmed fears.

Conclusion...

Every success story, every great leader, inventor, writer, and spiritual guru had one thing in common—they had to overcome procrastination. Procrastination is a tool of the comfort zone to keep us stuck in a life-loop of chasing our tails. Procrastination is the resistance we feel when we finally step out and make a decision to better ourselves. To defeat procrastination is simple but it does not mean it is easy. If your actions are causing you to feel anxiety, worry, or fear, and if they are making those around you uncomfortable, that is GOOD. It means you are on your way to creating your authentic life that is built by your standards.

Any of the dozen techniques will work when you feel that grasp of resistance. I wish you peace, love and inspiration on your journey.

Dream Big!

Bill Cortright
Miami, FL

Bibliography

Peale, Norman Vincent. "The Power of Positive Thinking," Simon & Schuster 1952

Dr. Hagelin, John. "Our body is really the product of our thoughts"

Dr. Dyer, Wayne. "I Can See Clearly Now," Hayhouse 2014

Hill, Napoleon. "Think and Grow Rich," Ralston Society 1937

Pressfield, Steven. "The War of Art," Black Irish Books 2002

Dr. Maxwell Maltz . "Psycho-Cybernetics," Prentice-Hall 1960

Segerstrom, Suzanne. Psychologist at University of Kentucky Curriculum Vitae 1999

Dr. McGonigal, Kelly. "The Willpower Instinct" Avery 2011

Ph.D Hanson, Rick Neuropsychologist Founder of The WellSpring Institute for Neuroscience and Contemplative Wisdom

Cuddy, Amy. Harvard Social Psychologist with Carney, Dana Berkley experiment "The Power of Power Posing," Dash.Harvard.edu 2012

2009 Study at the University of Exter, U.K.

2010 Study at University of Virginia

Dr.Pennebaker, James. Researcher "Writing to Heal," The University of Texas at Austin

About the Author

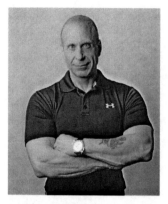

Bill Cortright is a highly sought after international speaker specializing in personal development, motivation, wellness, anti-aging, weight loss, and stress management. Bill's journey began like most at a young age struggling with weight loss/maintenance, resulting in a decade long fluctuation of 100 plus pounds three times before successfully losing the weight and eventually becoming a seven-time body-building champion. Today he is one of the top experts in the field of wellness, weight loss and stress management. Bill is the author of the international bestseller *The NEW Stress-Response Diet and Lifestyle Program* and has the soon to be released sequel called *The Seven Steps to Stress Mastery.*

Bill has spent three decades coaching clients from around the world with his cutting edge scientific approach to total wellness. This new and innovative approach is the result of Bill's personal experience of growing up obese and being diagnosed with diabetes. Bill realized that there was a major disconnect between the medical field and the diet and fitness industries. Patients are stressed, overwhelmed, tired, confused, depressed and frustrated. To create a real wellness plan everyone must work together and this has been the basis of Bill's work.

Bill's lectures speak from the heart of his personal experiences of battling diabetes and obesity but also from his profound understanding how our body and mind work in creating a life of health and prosperity. Bill, now in his fifties has turned his attention to the unique needs of the body as we age and how to master our own genetics through lifestyle management. Bill's new book *The Seven Steps to Stress Mastery* will address the science to the spiritual effects of managing stress. His mission is to motivate, educate and inspire people to live their best lives. Bill is resides in Miami, Florida with his wife, Linda and dogs, Toby and Charlie, and remains devoted to his family and his work.

Free Course: Living in the Green Zone

TRUTH: The Ten-Minute Life Plan, Ending Procrastination and Creating the Life You Want, is based off the science of how our body and nervous system handles stress. The discovery of this will-power switch has changed my life and thousands of clients around the world that I work with.

The *Ten-Minute* book has given you a dozen techniques that will end procrastination in your life. I wanted to add something extra for you, so I created this course *"Living in the Green Zone."* The course consists of Five Videos that take you through each of the Five Life Categories: Career, Finance, Health, Relationships, Personal/Spiritual Development. Each category has its own video packed with information and tips to live in the Green Zone.

This course is absolutely free to everyone who has purchased this book. Simply visit: www.LivingRightWithBillCortright.com/10-minute-book

You may also join us and register for new e-books that are geared toward Stress Mastery at www.LivingRightWithBillCortright.com and join me Monday through Friday on "The Stress Mastery Podcast" which can be downloaded on all platforms or at www.TheStressMasteryPodcast.com.

I also invite you to connect with us on social media and join our private Facebook Group "The Stress Mastery Podcast" https://www.facebook.com/groups/632834633571980/

Connect with Us

Facebook: Bill Cortright
https://www.facebook.com/bill.cortright.92

Twitter: @BillCortright
https://twitter.com/BillCortright

The Stress Mastery Podcast: iTunes
https://itunes.apple.com/us/podcast/stress-mastery-podcast-living-right-billcortright/
id1212468485?mt=2

Instagram: @livingrightwithbillcortright
https://www.instagram.com/livingrightwithbillcortright/

Emails:
Info for website, podcast and general information:
Info@livingrightwithbillcortright.com

To Contact Bill Directly:
Bill@livingrightwithbillcortright.com

For business development, website design and podcast production:
David@livingrightwithbillcortright.com

For information on speaking:
Darlene@livingrightwithbillcortright.com

Visit Bill at www.LivingRightWithBillCortright.com
Twitter: @BillCortright
Facebook: Living Right with Bill Cortright
Email: Bill@LivingRightWithBillCortright.com

#stayinspired

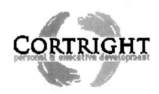

Index

CPSIA information can be obtained
at www.ICGtesting.com
Printed in the USA
LVOW10s0411310517

536363LV00011B/167/P